Be Your Best Body

Be Your Best Body™

*Every Woman's Fitness Guide to a
Strong and Graceful Body*

featuring

The Tone-Up™ *System*

by

Suesan Lazarus Pawlitski

*photographs by
Melanie Brickman Uranitsch*

Be Your Best Body™

Every Woman's Fitness Guide to a Strong and Graceful Body
featuring
The TONE-UP™ *System*

DISCLAIMER

Before beginning this, or any other, exercise program, it is advisable to obtain the approval and recommendations of your physician. This program is intended for people of all ages in good physical health. The purpose of this book is to educate and entertain. The author and TONE-UP Publishing shall have neither liability nor responsibility to any person or entity with respect to any loss or damage caused, or alleged to be caused, directly or indirectly by the information contained in this book.

If you do not wish to be bound by the above, you may return this book to the publisher for a full refund.

Text copyright © 1999 by Suesan Lazarus Pawlitski
Edited by Sydne Matus
Photographs © 1998 by Melanie Brickman Uranitsch
Model: Suesan Lazarus Pawlitski
Book and Cover Design by David Folkman
Audio Tape Music © 1998 by Jeff Elliot
Audio Tape Production by Mark DeAnda

Library of Congress Cataloging-in-Publication Data
Pawlitski, Suesan Lazarus
    Be Your Best Body: Every Woman's Fitness Guide to a Strong and Graceful Body
    featuring the TONE-UP System: by Suesan Lazarus Pawlitski
    p. cm.
    ISBN 0-9668504-2-4
    1. Exercise   2. Women's Health
    I. Pawlitski, Suesan Lazarus II. title
    Library of Congress Catalog Card Number: 98-96920

Published by:
    TONE-UP Publishing   **TONE-UP**
    P.O. Box 30058
    Santa Barbara, Ca. 93130, U.S.A.
    ToneUpPub@aol.com

    First Edition

10 9 8 7 6 5 4 3 2 1

Dedication

To my parents, Mell and Eileen,
who always encouraged me to follow my dreams no matter
how foolish they may have seemed.

Dad,
You are my mentor and I would have
never written this without your support.

To Garry, Briana and Tommy,
my loving husband and children,
thanks for believing in me.

In Memory of my Mother

Many thanks

for all your encouragement and help
in making this project come to life.
Mark Anthony, Nanette Boyer, Cathie Carr, Helen Curhan,
Mark DeAnda, Johnny Ebadi, Jeff Elliot, Barton Emmet,
Cynthia Emmet, David Folkman, Laurence Hauben,
Megan Kitchen, Mell Lazarus, Sally Mitchell Lazarus,
Sydne Matus, Mike Nichols, Susan Painter, Garry Pawlitski,
Dan Poynter, Merrily Smith, Melanie Brickman Uranitsch,
and Margie White.

Special thanks

to all my students and clients who have trusted me, taught me,
learned and laughed with me. Each of you has made a
difference in my life.

(This is a very abbreviated list of names, so if I left you out, I apologize.)

Ade, Adine, Al, Alan, Amanda, Anastasha, Andrea, Angie, Ann, Anna,
Annick, Antoinette, Araceli, Ariana, Barbara, Barbra, Bernadette, Betty,
Beverly, Bonnie, Bryn, Buffy, Carla, Carol, Carrie, Caryn, Cathy, Cecelia,
Ceci, Chelsea, Charlene, Chris, Christine, Christy, Cia, Cinda, Cindy, Clara,
Corrine, Cynthia, Dan, Dani, Dawn, Deanna, Debbie, Deborah, Debra, Diana,
Dick, Donna, Dorothy, Dotty, Ed, Ellen, Emily, Evonne, Fredda, Gaby, Gayle,
Gianna, Gigi, Gladys, Gretchen, Hala, Hallie, Harla, Heidi, Inge, Jaima, Jan,
Janet, Jean, Jenna, Jermaine, Jessica, Joan, JoAnn, John, Jonee, Josie, Joyce,
Judith, Judy, Julie, Julietta, June, Karen, Karsen, Kate, Kathleen, Kathryn,
Kathy, Katie, Keiko, Kelly, Kerri, Kerstin, Kim, Kirsten, Kit, Kristin,
Laurence, Laurie, Lane, Laura, Lauren, Lee, Lesley, Leslie, Libby,
Linda, Lisa, Lonna, Louise, Lucy, Lydia, Marea, Marguerita, Marie,
Mariette, Marilyn, Marlen, Marla, Marta, Mary, Maze, Megan, Melanie,
Melody, Meredith, Mia, Michele, Michelle, Monica, Muriel, Nancy, Nanette,
Naomi, Norma, Pam, Pamela, Pat, Patti, Penny, Phoebe, Priscilla, Rachael,
Randy, Rita, Rebecca, Rene, Robert, Robyn, Roxie, Sally, Sandy, Sara,
Sharon, Sheila, Sheri, Shirley, Solange, Susan, Sue, Suzy, Tara, Terry,
Thia, Timi, Toni, Trudi, Tybie, Victoria, Virginia, Walter, Yvonne.

Table of Contents

ABC's of TONE-UP

Alternate, Breathe, Check your posture
Deeper and wider, an Exact science
Firm and flat . . . Good!
Heels up, Intense
Just eight more times!
Kind classmates, (kinky jokes)
Last eight, really . . .
My we work hard . . . never enough reps.
Only four more times . . . don't believe it!
Plie, Quality workout
Results, results, results . . .
Sisters in suffering! Shhhhh . . .
Tight abs, Ultimate toning, Vibrant muscles
Walking in place, Xtra strong women!
Youthful attitudes, Zestful bodies.

by Ade Winger
TONE-UP Devotee

Chapter 1

Excuses, Excuses, No More Excuses!

The wise woman is capable of doing anything she wants, but doesn't feel she has to prove it. There may never be a reason to move your own furniture, change a tire, or mow the lawn, but it sure would be nice to know that you could if you had to!

And what about the high likelihood of having to carry your own groceries, or the certainty of having to get up from a chair.

Imagine your future. The fastest-growing age group in the United States is sixty-five and older. The biggest fear among that age group is not being able to maintain the lifestyle they are used to. If you don't take care of yourself now, the option of being independent and able to do simple tasks may not be there later.

Ask anyone who's become dependent on others. She feels like a terrible burden. Hopefully you and I will never be in that situation.

Regular exercise can improve or maintain your health and capabilities. It's a key factor in growing old gracefully. Now is the time to put yourself first. It's your responsibility to your family and friends to take care of yourself.

So often, I'll be at the grocery store, doing errands, or out to dinner and I'll run into someone who confesses to me that she hasn't been exercising. The fact that I instill guilt doesn't thrill me, but it has exposed me to a whole range of excuses people use. Maybe one or two of these will sound familiar to you.

- ▶ I'm too old.
- ▶ I have to get into shape first.
- ▶ I have no energy for exercise.
- ▶ I'm too fat; I need to lose weight first.
- ▶ I don't want to get bulky muscles like a bodybuilder.
- ▶ If I stop exercising, my muscles will turn to flab.
- ▶ I'm menopausal, (or prenatal, pregnant, postpartum,)
- ▶ My doctor told me not to exercise.
- ▶ My doctor said I may need to have surgery soon.
- ▶ I'm just too busy.

If one or more of these sound familiar, hopefully you'll see the light. There are no excuses.

Too old? Not in good enough shape? No energy?

You can increase your muscle mass and strength at any age and any time. If you don't use a muscle, it atrophies: It degenerates and becomes weaker. Remember the admonition "Use it or lose it?" Well, it's true.

Muscle growth, or hypertrophy, is the only way to raise your metabolism, which transforms your body into a more efficient machine. The more muscle you have, the more calories you utilize with every movement. You have more energy to burn when you're fit.

2

If you don't exercise, you lose muscles, your bones become less dense, and your metabolism drops. Then you become sluggish and the pounds slowly but surely pile on over the years. It has nothing to do with age, only with lack of exercise.

Exercise physiologist Daniel Rooks, a researcher at Beth Israel Hospital and an instructor in medicine in the Division on Aging at Harvard Medical School, conducted a study on fourteen women, aged 60 to 77. They participated in three one-hour strength-training sessions per week for sixteen weeks. They did lower- and upper-body exercises on machines. They used no cardiovascular equipment. At the end of the four months, the women's isotonic strength (which is needed to lift groceries, for instance) increased an average of 52 percent, and their isometric strength (needed to do things like get up from a chair) rose by 31 percent. In addition, their walking speed increased by 18 percent.

About these findings, Dr. Rooks said, "They show that proper conditioning translates into an improved ability to perform daily activities that are critical to maintaining independence."

> "Where would I be . . . What would I be . . . without TONE-UP?? It keeps me energized and has reshaped my body by firming my legs and arms. I have been told I look great in my skirts from behind!
>
> My goal is to be a TONE-UP user the rest of my life and as my grandchildren get older I will still be able to keep up with them or . . . better yet . . . have them keep up with me!!"
>
> —*Harla Hampton, 54 years young*
> *7 years of TONE-UP*

Too Fat? Want to drop those pounds first?

Exercise helps you lose weight. Sure, you may feel the need to lose a few

3

> "Since I began taking TONE-UP I have become much stronger. I could barely do one full body push-up and now I can do twenty-five! I have more energy and stamina. I have more endurance with my aerobic activities. My body has more muscle definition and I feel great. It has been a great confidence builder. When complete strangers stop me in the grocery store and tell me how fit I look, I think to myself, 'It's really working!'"
>
> *—Antoinette Campanelli, age 37*
> *8 years of TONE-UP*

pounds first, but you may be defeating the purpose if you don't combine exercise with dieting. Dieting alone results in a loss of half muscle—half fat.

When diet is combined with exercise, you decrease your percentage of body fat while maintaining, or increasing, your muscle mass which results in major proportional changes. Instead of ending up as a thinner version of what you were, you could reshape your figure as you slim down. You may as well do both at the same time.

Afraid of bulk or flab?

Women's genetic makeup generally keeps us from getting bulky. Believe it or not, it takes a lot of hard work to look like a bodybuilder! In the unlikely case that you wake up one morning with big, bulky muscles, you'll find that if you just stop the program you've been doing, they'll disappear very quickly.

Flab is synonymous with fat. Muscle and fat are two completely separate things; therefore, muscle cannot turn into flab. When you stop exercising, your muscles atrophy, so you have relatively more fat. That's the flabby part.

Menopausal? Pregnant? Postpartum?

Because we go through so many changes during menopause, e.g., hot flashes,

4

irregular periods, and emotional ups and downs, regular exercise may be the only consistent part of our lives. With a life expectancy of about eighty years old, we could expect to live almost forty percent of our lives after menopause.

"I took TONE-UP throughout my entire pregnancy and it en-abled me to control my weight and stay energized. I strongly encourage anyone to try it."
—*Katherine Boone, age 34*
2 years of TONE-UP

Two of the major risks associated with menopause are osteoporosis, a rapid, painless loss of bone mass, and cardiovascular disease, which includes heart attacks and strokes.

"At a time when my friends are having serious back trouble I have never felt stronger or straighter."
—*Joan Watson, age 57*
3 years of TONE-UP

The UC Berkeley Wellness Letter reports: "The more bone you build early in life, the better you will be able to withstand bone loss later. But even if you've waited until your forties, fifties, or sixties, there's still plenty of reason to follow this preventive program: 1) Make weight-bearing exercise part of your daily life, 2) consume enough calcium, 3) if you smoke, stop, 4) if you drink, drink only lightly or moderately, and 5) consider hormone replacement therapy."

"I recently had a bone density test and the results were above normal for my age group. Those results were particularly impressive because my mother suffered from severe arthritis, plus I have a predisposition for osteoporosis because of my slight frame, light skin and eyes. I am lactose intolerant which has prevented me from using milk products for the past five years.

I attribute my skeletal health to TONE-UP, a 'weight-bearing' class."
—*Nancy Panizzon, age 54*
10 years of TONE-UP

The TONE-UP system includes weight-bearing exercises which strengthen your muscles, bones, and heart.

TONE-UP is safe for women who plan to get pregnant, are pregnant, and those who never intend to get pregnant. Of course, before beginning an exercise program, it's wise to get your doctor's okay.

Your doctor said not to exercise?

Unless you have a very specific injury, ailment, or disease, perhaps you should start interviewing new doctors.

Granted, some forms of exercise may be hazardous to your health, like deep sea diving, hang-gliding, football, and motor-cross racing, but my TONE-UP system is a very safe and grounded form of exercise. The risk factors are quite low, and if you need to check with your physician first, show him or her this book before you begin.

Planned surgery?

Of course it depends on what type of surgery you're having, but exercising

"I joined TONE-UP between two hip surgeries, four months apart. I began going to TONE-UP twice a week, and I noticed my legs getting stronger, but was shocked at the post surgical results! It was much easier to get off the toilet and to transfer in and out of bed—two of the most painful parts of hip recovery, as you are lifting your body with only one leg.

Another bonanza was to learn that I could stand balanced in the shower, rather than clutching onto a grab bar continually. I could also sit in chairs without having to carry a pillow around with me.

My physician, my physical therapist, and my friends notice the improvement, and give full credit to TONE-UP. I'm delighted that I got involved at such a critical time in my life."

—*Marlen Tilford,*
Senior Citizen
6 months of TONE-UP

pre-surgery can only help with your post-operative recuperation. When you are in good condition, your lungs can clear quicker, your muscles and bones heal quicker, and your overall strength is better.

Lack of time? We all have the same amount of time, but we don't always prioritize its use well.

There are 8,760 hours in a year, but knowing how difficult it is to find a few for yourself, I've come up with some ideas:

- Tell your staff you have an important meeting.
- Order a take-out dinner.
- Cut out an hour of television a day.
- Let your machine answer your phone.
- Have the kids clean their own rooms.
- Work only the hours you are paid for.

And, finally, my personal favorite:

- Get up one hour earlier. There are plenty of advantages to that. The phone isn't ringing, everyone's asleep, and there are *no* interruptions. It could even become your favorite time of the day!

Your mind is a powerful thing. Use it positively and develop self discipline. Make your workout time a priority and don't let anyone or anything get in the way.

> "I have been taking TONE-UP two to three times per week for the last ten years. I feel it has given me the strength and flexibility to easily move from one athletic sport to another."
> —*Donna Waggoner, age 49 years old*
> *10 years of TONE-UP*

Excuses, Excuses, No More Excuses!

Chapter 2

You Need Some Reasons? I'll Give You Reasons

- ▶ TONE-UP reshapes and tones your body.
- ▶ TONE-UP improves posture.
- ▶ TONE-UP improves balance and coordination.
- ▶ TONE-UP increases energy.
- ▶ TONE-UP develops muscular strength.
- ▶ TONE-UP increases muscular endurance.
- ▶ TONE-UP improves stamina.
- ▶ TONE-UP increases flexibility.
- ▶ TONE-UP increases metabolism.
- ▶ TONE-UP improves sleep.
- ▶ TONE-UP helps prevent osteoporosis.
- ▶ TONE-UP may decrease incidence of hot flashes.
- ▶ TONE-UP improves injury recovery.
- ▶ TONE-UP burns lots of calories.
- ▶ TONE-UP builds cardiovascular capacity
- ▶ TONE-UP increases cardiovascular endurance.

▸ TONE-UP decreases blood pressure.

▸ TONE-UP increases body awareness.

▸ TONE-UP increases ability to handle stress.

▸ TONE-UP improves self-image.

▸ TONE-UP makes everyday activities easier.

▸ TONE-UP improves athletic performance.

▸ TONE-UP improves circulation.

▸ TONE-UP improves mood.

▸ TONE-UP makes you look and feel better.

▸ TONE-UP helps maintain ideal body weight.

▸ TONE-UP is better than the alternative!

Why do I do TONE-UP?

▸ To keep up with my kids.

▸ So I will always look younger than my husband.

▸ So my thin clothes still fit.

▸ To hear people say, "You look like you work out."

▸ Because I love to eat.

▸ To maintain my excellent health and quality of life.

▸ It's good for me.

▸ And for all the above reasons.

▸ Because I love the results and I know it works!

Chapter 3

A Little Quiz

Before we get to the really good stuff, let's see how much you already know. Here's a little quiz for you to take right now and then again after you've read the book, where you'll find all the answers.

Answer True or False

(answers to quiz page 114)

	T	F
1. The wise woman is one who is able to do anything she wants, but doesn't have to prove it.	☐	☐
2. Aging is the only reason our muscles get weaker.	☐	☐
3. Only aerobic exercise increases your metabolism.	☐	☐
4. Muscle can turn to flab.	☐	☐
5. Osteoporosis and cardiovascular disease are two major risks associated with menopause.	☐	☐
6. There are no good excuses for not doing the TONE-UP system.	☐	☐

Answer True or False

	T	**F**

7. There's a lot more to proper exercise than just lifting weights. ☐ ☐

8. To be truly fit you need to incorporate training in strength, endurance, balance, coordination, and flexibility. ☐ ☐

9. TONE-UP is a no-bulk form of exercise. ☐ ☐

10. The stronger you become the less you need to challenge yourself. ☐ ☐

11. After two weeks of exercise your body begins to change physically. ☐ ☐

12. Suesan's primary concern is to make sure that her clients are receiving quality instruction, information, and care, and are achieving results. ☐ ☐

13. Muscles don't grow old, they just get lazy. ☐ ☐

14. A balanced diet consists of protein, fat and carbohydrates. ☐ ☐

15. A healthy weight loss is five pounds a week. ☐ ☐

Answer True or False

	T	**F**
16. One gram of protein is equal to four calories.	☐	☐
17. One gram of fat is equal to 3,500 calories.	☐	☐
18. Eating less than 1,200 calories a day will slow down the weight-loss process.	☐	☐
19. Muscle weighs more than fat.	☐	☐
20. The best way to measure your fitness progress is to weigh yourself on a scale.	☐	☐
21. Sleeping is an aerobic activity.	☐	☐
22. Drinking water while you exercise will cause cramping and nausea.	☐	☐
23. Genetics is 100% responsible for your shape.	☐	☐
24. Chest and buttocks are opposing muscle groups.	☐	☐
25. Static stretching is a bouncing movement.	☐	☐

Answer True or False

	T	F
26. The most important part of your body, aside from your head, is your torso.	☐	☐
27. Neutral alignment is relative to the room you're in.	☐	☐
28. Your old tennis shoes are perfect for TONE-UP.	☐	☐

Chapter 4

Principles of the Tone-Up™ System

Are you willing to form a new habit that can improve your life and allow you to live up to your own physical potential? Ready to reshape yourself into your best body? If you answered yes, then you're in the right place.

Thanks for choosing the TONE-UP system. And, congratulations for taking responsibility for yourself, because it means you're willing to make your own best choices. Selecting my system is the best choice.

Why is a *system* so important? It's true, you'd get some results from doing biceps curls and bench presses, but they may not be the results you want. There's a lot more to proper exercise than just lifting weights.

"Suesan's TONE-UP class is an excellent vehicle for women to gain strength all over. She targets every muscle group, and with her training knows exactly how one should posture one's self while performing each movement. Well-balanced body strength creates a wonderful side-effect of confidence and well-being, as well as the obvious—better physical performance in sports."

—*Chris Robinson, age 47*

To sculpt a single muscle is simple, but reshaping a whole body is another matter.

This is where the ᴛᴏɴᴇ-Uᴘ system comes in.

It's a finely tuned exercise program that has evolved over the past 15 years. It combines physiologically sound and effective exercises that I've developed from ballet, modern dance, Pilates principles, yoga, weight room workouts, and calisthenics.

"ᴛᴏɴᴇ-Uᴘ's leg work has come in handy while visiting third world countries!"
—*Evonne Dicus,*
age 59
5 years of ᴛᴏɴᴇ-Uᴘ

The exercises alternate from toning to strengthening techniques and are designed to develop the elongated muscles of a dancer as opposed to the compact muscles of a bodybuilder. This is a *no-bulk workout.* By following the program in its specific, logical order, you will progress comfortably from one exercise to the next.

I'll remind you repeatedly about correct body alignment and proper technique so that you achieve the maximum benefits from each exercise.

With improved posture, your body will not only appear longer and leaner, but your muscles will become equally and proportionately balanced. With the added use of resistance from light weights and

"When I found ᴛᴏɴᴇ-Uᴘ, a year and a half ago, I was excited to find a workout that encompassed the fundamentals of many physical disciplines that I had learned throughout my life; ballet, modern dance, yoga, weight training and various aerobic methods.

Along with that, Suesan's methods are perpetually evolving making one's goals attainable while at the same time pushing you to set new ones. It's a very creative form of exercise and a GREAT workout!"
—*Andrea Beloff, age 33*
1 and a half years of ᴛᴏɴᴇ-Uᴘ

gravity, you will improve your muscle strength, endurance, balance, coordination, and agility.

Let's begin by looking at the present. Is your lifestyle allowing you to do all you want to in life? Are you in good enough condition to join your friends for an impromptu ski weekend? Play eighteen holes of golf? Go out dancing? Play doubles tennis? Participate in a walk-a-thon with your kids or grandkids?

To be truly fit, you need to incorporate training in strength, endurance, balance, coordination and flexibility. Skiing, golf, tennis, and walking, individually, do not develop all these factors.

First become fit and then you can excel at sports and enjoy them more. Being a weekend athlete is potentially injurious. We all know people who work at a sedentary job all week long and then squeeze in all their recreation on the weekend. By Monday, they are either so sore they can barely move or are nursing a pulled muscle.

What about all the repetitive-motion and work-related injuries that are popping up all over the place? This book and workout concentrate on how to be aware and become conscious of your body alignment at all times. Carpal tunnel syndrome, tennis elbow, rotator cuff, and lower back pain can all be minimized or prevented through both your consciousness and the correctly aligned stretching and strengthening exercises provided with Tone-Up.

Do you want to lose weight? Tone-Up increases your metabolism which causes you to burn more fat and calories.

> "As a result of my Tone-Up workouts my muscles stay strong and toned, allowing me to continue playing competitive soccer with women half my age."
>
> —*Christy Kelso, age 45*
> *5 years of Tone-Up*

Your aerobic and anaerobic capacities will also improve allowing you to walk, run, hike, ski, and play sports longer without tiring out.

Looking and feeling good aren't always primarily weight dependent. How you present yourself is a large part of how you appear. By improving your posture, muscle balance, and tone you may realize that weight wasn't your problem.

This first book represents the foundation of the Tone-Up system. Although the information is basic, the workout is geared toward all levels of fitness and it's up to you how hard or easy you'd like to make it.

> "What would I do without my Tone Up video???? I moved back to France five years ago with my family after 20 years of California life and 15 years of almost daily exercise with Suesan where I got introduced to the many merits of Tone-Up. It is a wonderful whole body workout.
>
> I now slip Suesan's video into the VCR, open all the windows wide (we're right on the breakwater of a tiny fishing village) and do Tone-Up. It gives me back that great sense of good posture and muscle tone. Doing it regularly makes my muscles stronger and more supple.
>
> So I guess it's Tone-Up for life! I now know the tape by heart of course, but I still put it on for the company and the encouragement..."
>
> —*Annick Lee, age 53,*
> *10 years of Tone-Up*
> *Ciboure, Basque country, France*

My Advice

The most important piece of advice I can offer you is: *Listen*.

1. *Listen to all of my instructions* and safety tips. Pretend that I'm standing right beside you. Take everything I say personally, because listening carefully will lessen any risk of injury.

2. *Listen to your body*. If an exercise produces a slight burning sensation or shaking of your muscles, that's good. Your goal is to have to stop and rest because you're working hard.

Check and recheck your form and alignment to see if you are doing the exercise correctly. If you get any joint pain, you need to decide whether or not to do that particular exercise. Maybe the resistance you have chosen is too heavy right now. In any case, you have plenty of opportunities to stop, reassess the exercise, and then resume the program.

I believe the most important factor in any exercise program is *quality* rather than *quantity*. Your first goal is to master the form and your second is to increase the intensity. As you get more comfortable with the exercises, you *then* add either more repetitions or weight so you are constantly challenging and improving yourself.

"In my mid-thirties I took Tone-Up to look good. And there is no doubt that Tone-Up works your figure into great shape. But, over the years my commitment vacillated and, like many working moms, my needs got sidelined too easily.

Today, I realize that Tone-Up is the ideal exercise program to attain robust health. It combines ballet moves with weight bearing and stretching techniques that strengthen my body from head to toe. After a workout my body is tingling with endorphins (natural) and my energy level is sky high.

Because of my renewed commitment to Tone-Up and myself I am able to do all the things in life that mean the world to me: Gardening, walking, horseback riding, and living harmoniously with my body, mind and spirit."

—*Cathy Fletcher, age 46*
2 solid years of Tone-Up

Completing this program two to three times a week, to the best of your ability, guarantees positive changes in your body in as soon as six weeks. Combining this program with a healthy diet and some aerobic activities will accelerate the process and successfully get you on your way to a healthy, active lifestyle.

Before you get started, I suggest that you read this entire book. It is crucial to look over all the photographs and descriptions so your form is correct. Read Chapter 10 carefully so you understand how and why we're doing it this way. Also, it is a good idea to get your doctor's approval before undertaking any exercise program.

On the chance that you never read this introduction again, I will thank you in advance for once again proving Tone-Up a success!

Chapter 5

What to Expect and How to Set Realistic Goals

Let's be realistic. Start exercise moderately. Don't expect the impossible from yourself. Feeling and looking better won't happen in one day.

Be patient. Remember, you didn't get into the your present shape overnight. You need to start out with TONE-UP two to three times a week, and keep in mind the Four Stages of Becoming An Exerciser (see below). If you are consistent, and keep challenging yourself, you will see progress very soon.

Most important, make realistic goals and stick to them. Make TONE-UP a part of your life.

What to Expect In as short as two weeks of TONE-UP, your body will begin to change *physiologically*. You'll feel stronger and your muscle endurance will increase.

"Even though Suesan's TONE-UP class is probably the most vigorous class I've ever taken, it definitely has provided the most beneficial results in my sports activities. I am able to play 3-4 sets of tennis without feeling utterly exhausted afterwards. In addition the class is a great conditioner for hiking up hills, walking and biking. And lastly, I feel good and am keeping fit!"
—*Gladys Robinson, Senior Citizen*
7 months of TONE-UP

At six weeks, your body will begin to change *physically*. You'll notice positive changes in your muscle tone and overall appearance. This is when the compliments start coming your way. Your friends will wonder if you lost weight, got a new hair style, or are wearing a new outfit. They'll know something's up, but aren't quite sure what it is.

By now, you're seeing improvements. You're thinking, "I've been doing this for six weeks, and finally, it's starting to get easier." This is when you should increase your repetitions and/or your weights. The point is, you don't want it to get easier!

Exercise is a series of challenges designed to fulfill your fitness goals. You need to push yourself beyond your comfort zone.

Make it worth your while. Let me explain.

The Four Stages of Becoming an Exerciser

1. The Baby Stage
You're confused and trying to figure out what you're supposed to be doing. Everything is new to you. Your mind is willing but your body's not able. You feel some frustration, but you keep on trying.

2. The Toddler Stage

Your muscles are developing and you're beginning to realize you're in charge of your own destiny. You're determined to learn and do it right. You're ready to accept all challenges. You now see that the rewards are worth the effort.

3. The Teenage Stage

You think you know just about everything you need to know. Nobody is going to tell you how to do it any better or differently. You've reached a fitness plateau. You're bored; apathy sets in. You decide that you've reached the epitome and you're now just going along for the ride. Don't get stuck in this stage!

4. The Adult Stage

This is a great place to be! You've realized that you're still capable of learning. You don't know it all. You're ready for new challenges and can push yourself a little further. Your potential is unlimited. You no longer depend on someone else to "give you a good workout."

Keep in mind that the stronger you become, the quicker your muscles feel what they are supposed to feel.

For example, when you first start doing lunges, you will feel them just about anywhere and everywhere from your hips

"TONE-UP has helped to heal my injured knee by building up my leg muscles. I am now able, for the first time ever, to get a quick aerobic workout by going up and down 241 stair steps to the beach three consecutive times! And I feel great!!"

—*Ellen Downing, age 69*
6 months of TONE-UP

23

down. And, that's okay. But eventually you will be able to isolate exactly which muscles you are working, and you'll feel your thigh and buttock muscles working right away. That's a good thing. It means your muscles are getting smarter.

This is the time for you to decide the fate of your body. It's never too late. Muscles don't grow old, they just get lazy! As long as you're going to live a long time, you may as well be your best body.

"For many years all I did was running and aerobics. TONE-UP, my tune-up class, is what changed my muscle build and stamina. It is a complete physical and mental workout requiring a full mind-body connection. I believe that all the plies, squats and weight training are an investment in my body's health.

The most challenging part of the class is staying focused and making all the tiny little adjustments to make the workout work for you. But, even that becomes easy when you have Suesan as an instructor."

—*Leslie Somma, age 31*
5 years of TONE-UP

Chapter 6

Meet Your Teacher

You may be wondering, "Who is this woman I'm willing to trust with my body?" Well, I'm not a model, an actress, a fitness superstar, or even a famous author. But I am a teacher. A deeply committed teacher.

My goal as a teacher is to educate my students how to understand and reach the full potential of their bodies, without placing unnecessary demands upon themselves. I strive to make exercise a rewarding and enjoyable experience. Functional fitness, which helps make daily tasks simpler, should be a part of everyone's life. It's an integral part of attaining and maintaining good health and function, as well as achieving longevity.

On a personal level, I get incredible joy and satisfaction from teaching. I learn from my students that there are more reasons to stay fit than I ever imagined. Throughout this

"Suesan's TONE-UP program is brilliant! I am not naturally athletic and do not love to exercise. But Suesan continues to inspire me; she makes me want to work out. She knows how to push one to work hard and safely, without injury.

TONE-UP has completely changed my body in terms of appearance, energy and stamina, and my back troubles have disappeared. I was never able to stick with any exercise program until this one."
—*Nancy Kawalek, ageless*
6 years of TONE-UP

book, you are reading some real-life testimonials, and I'm sure you will find some relevant to you.

I get concerned when I see someone become overly fanatical about how much exercise she gets or how little she eats to attain a certain look. If she normally exercises daily and then feels guilty for missing a single workout, that's a bit much.

I express to my clients that it's more important to be consistent, continually challenge yourself, and practice moderation.

Prevention of injuries and improper use is important. Of course it depends on one's goals. A competitive athlete may need to take some risks to achieve her goals,

> "I find TONE-UP to be a great support to my overall fitness, especially in the areas of strength and flexibility. The classes are challenging and offer a balance to my workout regime by educating me to the concepts of alignment, isolation, strength building and stretching.
>
> I know that this knowledge and conditioning contributed to my staying healthy and for the most part injury free during more than 8 years of sports competition.
>
> Suesan's thoughtful design of the class and skill in explaining and educating, have taught me a great deal about my body and how to take care of it.
>
> I can honestly say that TONE-UP has made a difference in how my body feels, looks and works for me."
>
> —*Michele Pezzoli, age 49*
> *13 years of TONE-UP*

but, if the objective is feeling and looking better, risks simply aren't worth taking.

I teach exercise classes thirteen hours a week, which, I consider a bit excessive. But when I teach, I don't do everything that I have my classes do (but don't tell them that), plus I've built up to teaching that many over several years. My weekly teaching schedule consists of ten TONE-UP classes and three low-impact aerobics, and that's plenty for me.

I don't run, hike, in-line skate, ski, cycle or even garden on a regular basis. But when I do an activity, I don't get sore and I'm strong enough to keep up the pace.

I feel like a couch potato compared to some other fitness professionals whose videos, books and interviews I've seen. Their lifestyles seem to me unrealistic and unreasonable. Sure, anyone can appear fit when she spends most of her life exercising and watching everything she eat. But, who has the time or even the desire?

Fitness wasn't always a big part of my life. In fact, my active social life was the most important part of my high school years. Academics came next and athletics were non existent. I used every excuse known to woman to get out of physical education classes. So how did I become a teacher?

The year was 1980. I began teaching exercise entirely by accident. I was a newly married college graduate with a degree in modern dance (I'll explain how I got there in the nutrition chapter). I wasn't an athlete or even a sports enthusiast. In fact, exercise was a forbidden word in the world of dance. We *moved*, not exercised, our bodies.

I moonlighted as a jazz and disco dance teacher (yes, disco) while working as a retail store manager. One day, completely bored with my full-time job, I phoned around town to see if anyone was hiring dance teachers.

A studio called Bodyfirm said they didn't offer dance

> "I have been taking TONE-UP classes with Suesan since before it was called TONE UP. This is the only system I find consistently productive and always challenging.
>
> I have acquired awareness of my own body and have never felt unnatural aches and pains afterwards. I know my body has become stronger and better aligned."
>
> —*Cynthia Emmet, age 71*
> *15+ years of TONE-UP*

but were looking for exercise instructors with dance training and teaching experience. They invited me to take a class and I decided to give it a try. I walked into a packed room of very fit woman who were executing, effortlessly, what felt like a jillion repetitions of leg lifts, jumping jacks, and side bends. I was in awe.

I guess all my performance training paid off, because I fooled them into thinking that I, too, was in great shape. They hired me on the spot!

What surprised me most about teaching exercise was the variety of people it attracted. Dancers lived, breathed, and talked dance, whereas these exercisers actually had lives outside the gym. They were entrepreneurs, employees, students, parents, professionals, and artists. However, they all shared a common goal, which was to look good. And these non-dancers did look good. I was now among people who moved to live, not lived to move.

The word aerobics had not come into use yet. We played our music on a record player. The dancing was twelve minutes of high kicks and knee lifts. Tennis shoes or no shoes were our choice of footwear.

We exercised primarily to maintain our body weight. We bounced, reached, and pushed our bodies in any possible way so we could "feel the burn." This program wasn't intended for anyone with weak knees, back, ankles, or heart. At twenty-five years old, fortunately, I was still pliable. If by thirty-five you weren't already in great condition, you could just hang up your tennis shoes!

Requirements for becoming an aerobics instructor included being able to kick higher than anyone else, count in eights, and holler instructions while maintaining some semblance of order behind you. The aim was to see how many students you could kill. It literally became "survival of the fittest!"

I enjoyed teaching but certainly didn't aspire to be an aerobics instructor forever. I was sure this was just a craze that would prove to be bad for our health and, therefore, end shortly. This was to be just a temporary job while I raised my young children. I was even embarrassed to tell people what I did for a living. I felt I would eventually get a "real job."

It's now the turn of the millennium, many years have passed, and my part-time job has long been my career. The aerobics-surviving baby boomers are now establishing the trends of the future. There are exercise options for everyone at any age or fitness level.

> "I have tried different exercise regimes over the past 25 years including lap swimming, tennis, weights, aerobics, and yoga.
>
> Then I found TONE-UP!
>
> When I went skiing this year, I had the stamina to continue skiing all day without stopping and panting every 15 minutes! In fact, I skied for three days straight and never got sore muscles! This was amazing to me . . . until I realized it was because of the strengthening and conditioning I have achieved from TONE-UP.
>
> TONE-UP is unsurpassed for localized muscle group conditioning. It lets no muscle go un-worked! The benefits reaped are noticeable. I highly recommend TONE-UP for anyone looking for an efficient, total body workout!"
>
> —*Barbra Mousouris, age 46*
> *1 year of TONE-UP*

Certification programs and higher education in Health and Fitness-related fields have raised the standards. Licensing could be in the near future. Even the Surgeon General warns us that the lack of exercise is dangerous to our health. Exercise has become a necessity rather than a diversion.

It's ironic that nowadays we need to make such an effort to exercise, when just a few decades ago people worked their bodies hard every day just to survive. Our ancestors milked the cows, tilled the soil, and washed their clothes by hand. Today, the idealized lifestyle includes hiring people to do these jobs. So, what do we do? We do exercises that simulate milking cows, tilling soil, and washing clothes by hand.

Apart from my husband, Garry, and my two teen-aged children, Briana and Tommy, TONE-UP brings me my greatest personal fulfillment. I take it very seriously. My primary commitment is to make sure that my clients are receiving quality instruction, information, and care, and are achieving results.

Allow me to be your personal trainer. I've made my commitment to guide you along. You simply need to follow this exercise system regularly, and you will realize the incredible potential you and your body have.

As we age we become more experienced, confident, and wise; why shouldn't we also become more energetic, strong, and healthy?

Nineteen years ago, I found myself in the right place at the right time. Who would ever have guessed?

Well, now you are, too!

Chapter 7

Understanding Basic Nutrition

*Written with the guidance of Nutritionist and
Diet Specialist Helen Curhan, M.P.H., R.D*

The basis for a balanced diet is elementary. You simply need to burn as many calories as you consume.

What a concept! Then why is food such an all-consuming obsession for so many of us? Especially when we're trying to lose weight?

What can I eat? When should I eat? Why am I eating at all? Do I need more protein, less fat? How many calories are too few? Too many?

Diet, according to Webster's dictionary, means *the food and drink regularly provided or consumed.* If that's all it is, why does that word cause so much anxiety? Why is it associated with self-deprivation and guilt?

A few years ago, I asked 300 women if they felt they were at their ideal weight. Six said yes, two wanted to gain a few pounds, but the overwhelming majority 292, wanted to lose weight. A few wanted to lose as much as fifty pounds but most believed that a two- to five-pound loss would make them feel better about themselves.

Even as a preteen and teenager, I was always trying to lose those last five pounds. I tried a variety of fad diets: e.g., Metrical, Ades Candies, Dexatrim, the Cabbage Soup Diet, the Grapefruit and Tuna Diet, the Liquid Protein Diet, and several more I can't even remember. I cut out starches, consumed high quantities of protein, gorged myself on carbohydrates, and ate all nonfat foods. I tested whatever was in at the time.

I remember getting inspired every few months to pump out 25 sit-ups and run in place for ten minutes before bedtime, and expecting to wake up the next morning five pounds lighter. My problem was that I was very inactive and out of shape. I expected miracles.

In college, I changed my major from elementary education to dance because I thought dancing seemed like fun, plus all the dancers looked so great. What could be better? I could earn a degree *and* get rid of those five extra pounds forever. Boy, was I wrong.

The dance classes were incredibly challenging and competitive, rehearsals were grueling, and performances were exhausting. Add to that the enormous emphasis on how we looked. Modern dance and ballet didn't keep us thin; the terrible eating habits did.

I was surrounded by eating disorders of all forms. Some dancers were addicted to diet soft drinks, chocolate, and cigarettes. Some were afraid to eat at all and became obsessed with their weight. I had one anorexic classmate who became so weak from malnutrition she was completely unable to dance. She sat in the corner, dressed in her baggy leotard, watching us with her sad, sunken eyes. I had never seen anyone like that before.

Well, that was then and this is now. Times have changed (or have they), and we've become more informed and smarter about the way we eat (or have we).

Is there any question in our minds as to why women are

still deluded that there are miracles diets and that dieting is the only way to lose weight?

We're exposed to it every day. Magazine covers highlight articles that are titled "Kiss 20 Pounds Goodbye," "Exercises to Lose Unsightly Cellulite," "Lose Those 10 Stubborn Pounds," and "52 Ways to Lose a Pound a Week."

We're still influenced by cover girls as role models. Eating disorders are at an all-time high, especially among young women. According to Pat Lyons, RN, MA (AFAA Fitness-Theory & Practice) "Last year Americans spent $30 billion on weight loss products and programs, including fitness programs. But statistics tell us that nine out of ten fail to maintain losses and risk their health in the process."

One sure way to fail at weight loss is by trying to lose weight too quickly. When you eat less than your body needs to run efficiently, you withdraw energy from your last meal. If your last meal didn't provide enough energy to sustain you, you'll begin to break down body fat and muscle, and through a few metabolic pathways you'll eventually begin to regain energy for your body. This will cause you to lose weight quickly.

"TONE-UP is the perfect balance between gentle yoga and rigorous aerobics. TONE-UP brims with good exercise: stretching, toning, balancing, light weight lifting. How can so much be accomplished by doing so little?

By attending TONE-UP twice a week and eating a sensible low-fat diet, I lost 14 lbs. over a 4-month period and looked and felt great."

—Sara Patchen,
52 years old
4 months of TONE-UP

This may sound good, but, the bad news is that if you use your muscles (lean tissue) for fuel, over time your metabolism slows down and you store more and more fat. This is *not* good.

In other words, cutting way down on the fuels you need by fasting and eating small quantities does not promote weight loss.

What is "less than your body needs to run efficiently?" The absolute minimum of calories that must be consumed daily is 1,200, and that's based on an inactive lifestyle. If you're not eating 1,200 calories a day, your body goes into starvation mode. Its biggest concern becomes where the next meal is coming from, and then everything eaten is stored as fat for survival purposes.

Fat keeps your body insulated and protects your organs. (Just in case you're ever lost in a snowstorm without food for a week, your body has the ability to store fat so you won't starve to death!)

Dieting, alone, results in loss of both fat and muscle.

Dieting plus exercise results in 100% fat loss and no muscle loss. If you lose weight while dieting and exercising, that means you are burning up stored fat.

Two pounds a week is a healthy weight loss. You know how weight sneaks up on you? Well, if you lose weight slowly, your body

"TONE-UP is a carefully crafted, muscle specific workout program. Participants are trained to work muscles safely, efficiently, and to maximum levels. The workout increases overall body strength, firms and tones muscle groups, helps to establish correct posture, and builds up ability to balance.

For me the best part is I feel fantastic, my friends say I look great, and my blue jeans fit! TONE-UP truly makes a difference in my life!!"

—*Ade Winger, age 51*

has a chance to adapt to the loss, and your chances of keeping it off will be better. Plus you're probably not torturing yourself with some radical diet.

We need to make becoming healthy our primary goal. New habits take time to make.

Think of your body as a car. You need fuel for the car to run. If you plan to travel far that day, you fill the car up. If you plan to leave the car in the garage for a day you don't need a whole lot of fuel in it.

There are seven basic nutrients essential for life. They are protein, carbohydrates, fats, fiber, vitamins, minerals, and water.

If you have a balance of proteins, carbohydrates, fats and water you will be receiving the fiber, vitamins and minerals needed.

Proteins   Proteins are made up of amino acids. The body needs twenty three amino acids which are essential and eight of them must be supplied from the diet. Our cells have the capacity to store amino acids so if you don't eat all that you need in a day, the amino acid pool allows the cells to release the stored amino acids into you system.

Proteins primarily build and repair body tissue since they are a structural part of every cell. They also make up hormones and enzymes in your body's neurotransmitters. They are an important component of our immune system.

Good sources of protein are tofu, soy beans, tempeh, nuts, seeds, poultry, fish, lean meats, and cheese (especially goat).

The essential amino acids are also provided by all nuts, sunflower and sesame seeds, peanuts, beans, carrots, bananas, brussels sprouts, cabbage, cauliflower, corn, cucumbers, eggplant, kale, okra, peas, potatoes, summer squash, sweet potatoes, and tomatoes.

There are four calories per one gram of protein.

Carbohydrates

Carbohydrates provide the best source of quick, short-term energy required, for example, when you run up a flight of stairs, lift a heavy bag of groceries, or get out of a car. Without carbohydrates you cannot utilize fats and proteins.

During the digestion of carbohydrates, they are broken down by water and enzymes into simple sugars. There is no discrimination by the body between complex and simple carbohydrates. They all become monosaccharides and glucose, which get absorbed into the bloodstream via the small intestine. These sugars are either burned as energy in the muscle or stored as fat. The consumption of carbohydrates drives the release of insulin, which is our fat-storing hormone.

The bottom line is: although they do make up the majority of a healthy diet, don't go overboard on them. If not utilized, they will store as fat. And fat is not utilized until the carbohydrates are depleted.

Beans, rice, potatoes, and whole grains are complex carbohydrates. Fruit and sugar are simple carbohydrates. As

> "After experiencing back and knee pain from my standard workout of running and climbing stadium steps, I decided to give TONE-UP a try. After just 3 months, I began to notice results. My back and knee pain were gone, and I felt stronger and more energized than ever. The program even encouraged me to reassess my eating habits. As a result, my clothes fit better and I consequently feel better about myself.
>
> Nine months later I still look forward to daily workouts. Without a doubt, Tone-Up has changed my life!"
>
> —*Cindy Taylor, 34 year old working mother*
> *9 months of TONE-UP*

explained above, they all assimilate as sugar, so don't forget to count them as calories if you are trying to lose weight.

There are four calories in one gram of carbohydrates.

Fats Fats protect internal organs and are a necessary part of each cell. The sex hormones are derived from a type of fat cholesterol, and so is cortisol, which is an important stress hormone.

Fat is a slower form of energy than carbohydrates and therefore the most efficient source of energy for sustained endurance activities.

Good sources of fats are those that are found in nuts, goat milk products, avocado, oils, olives, poultry, fish, and lean meats.

There are nine calories in one gram of fat.

The way you choose to eat is subjective. Whether you feel better physically or emotionally by eating properly or by giving into cravings of unhealthy foods, remember that you are in control of what you do. Your mind is more powerful than any cravings you may have. You only have one body and you need to take care of it.

In my relatively short life time, I have seen way too many people get sick, or die, of illnesses that are from poor lifestyle choices. I believe that what we consume, where we live, and how we spend our work and free time have a big effect on our ultimate outcome.

Eating good, natural, whole foods, and food combining, as outlined in "Fit For Life," by Harvey and Marilyn Diamond, make sense to me and fit into my lifestyle. I'm not always strict about what I eat, and enjoy treats as much as the next person, but I balance it out to make it as healthy as possible.

Eating Tips

▶ Don't assume that if it says nonfat, that you should eat it. Check what the main ingredients are. Often, non-fat foods are loaded with sugar, or carbohydrates to replace the fats.

▶ Watch for hidden sugars in ingredients: corn syrup, glucose, sucrose, maltose, and dextrose.

▶ Don't overeat. You'll gain weight.

▶ Eat as many vegetables as you can each day.

▶ Spread a little avocado on your sandwich instead of mayonnaise.

▶ Broccoli and bokchoy are great sources of calcium.

▶ Soybeans and tofu are excellent sources of protein.

▶ Edamames (soybean pods) make a tasty snack.

▶ An 8-ounce bag of potato chips has 80 grams of fat = 720 fat calories.

▶ Don't overeat. You'll feel sluggish.

▶ Don't skip breakfast.

▶ Drink at least eight glasses of water a day.

▶ Wait at least three hours between meals or snacks.

▶ Don't overeat. Eat more natural, whole foods if you're always hungry. They are more satiating than processed foods.

▶ Put grated carrots on your sandwiches. They moisten and sweeten the contents.

▶ Eat lots of high water foods, including vegetables and fruits.

▶ Always order salad dressing on the side. Lightly dip (not scoop) your fork into it, then into your salad.

▶ Don't overeat. Your body has to work too hard to digest all that food. Save your energy.

- ▶ Fresh is always best. Eat the real thing, including butter; not margarine.
- ▶ Darker vegetables generally have more nutrition.
- ▶ Avoid processed foods, and sugar and fat substitutes.
- ▶ All foods with warning labels should be avoided!
- ▶ If you crave something to eat, drink a big glass of water and wait twenty minutes. The craving should go away. Mind over matter! If you still crave it, then eat it before you eat everything else in the house.
- ▶ If you can't read it, don't eat it! Check ingredients.
- ▶ Don't overeat.
- ▶ Don't eat after 8 p.m. The last meal of your day needs three hours to digest before you go to bed. If your food is digested before you're asleep, all your energy can go into building and repairing your body.

Chapter 8

A Bit About Aerobic Exercise

"I just don't understand it," said Melissa with a sigh, as she sat eating her second nonfat muffin and drinking her nonfat cafe latte at the coffee house.

"I've cut out all fats and I certainly get lots of exercise. I play tennis twice a week, do my own gardening, plus just keeping up with my two-year old, you'd think I'd be skinny! Five years ago I was ten pounds lighter! I'm so frustrated. I'd do anything to lose some weight."

As she tilted her head back to drink the last sweet drops of her latte, she saw the clock on the wall.

"Oh, no! I've got to go. I've got a luncheon in an hour!"

We all know a Melissa, don't we? She has a misconception about diet, low-fat foods, and exercise, and it's time for her to try another plan of action. What would be the best changes for Melissa to make? Let's give her some advice. She says she wants to lose ten pounds and she'll do anything it takes.

For Melissa to safely lose ten pounds it could take her only five weeks if she cuts back her caloric intake to the minimum of 1,200 per day. Or she can cut back to 1,500 calories and burn an extra 300 calories daily.

41

Melissa can work it off however she wants, but she must either use more energy or consume 3,500 fewer calories for each pound she wants to lose.

TONE-UP two to three times a week will increase her metabolism, which will enable her to burn more calories and reshape her body. Adding aerobic exercise three times a week for twenty to sixty minutes will burn off stored fat.

Then, she needs to keep fit so the extra weight doesn't keep sneaking up on her. If she isn't willing to put that much aerobic exercise into her schedule, she'll still get great benefits from doing TONE-UP, reading my eating tips again, and improving her eating habits. It just may take a little longer, but it didn't all come on in one day either.

TONE-UP, along with aerobic exercise, will not only improve her tennis game and her attitude, it will also afford her less time to hang out in restaurants.

Let's say, hypothetically speaking, you are Melissa and you ask me to explain this "aerobics" thing. You think I'm going to tell you that you must do hours of dance-around-the-room-with-a-bunch-of-ladies every day in order to lose weight. Well, that's just not true. You could do any kind of aerobic activity that you enjoy to utilize stored fats in your body, and there are plenty of options.

Aerobic literally means "the body's ability to take in and use oxygen." To put it in simpler terms, when you exert a consistent, moderately intense amount of energy for twenty or more minutes, you use oxygen which fuels, or burns, fat as its main energy source.

You may think that aerobic exercise needs to be grueling. Actually, once you get past the first five to ten minutes it becomes a lot easier. Because you are using both fat and oxygen for energy, it's possible to endure aerobic exercise for a long period of time; for example, marathon running is an aerobic sport.

Why are the first five minutes of aerobic exercise the most difficult? This is the *anaerobic* portion which requires more glucose (sugar) and less fat. It is the adjustment period when you burn up your immediate energy sources which may make you feel winded and cause your muscles to burn. If you continue long enough at a pace that's not extremely taxing, your aerobic system will take over.

If you push yourself extremely hard, your anaerobic energy will become depleted and you will not be able to continue. A 100-yard dash is an anaerobic sport.

A typical day is primarily spent anaerobically, which means in shorter bursts of energy. Examples are, getting up off the couch, rushing to answer the phone, or going up a flight of

> "It constantly amazes me that after attending TONE-UP classes for many years now . . . they are never boring, it never feels too easy and its constantly challenging, I feel stronger. It's addicting (in a good way), and I look forward to it.
>
> I spent eight days in New York walking all day every day with my two sisters (one 4 years older and one 4 years younger) and while they were achy and tired I felt as if I could keep on going and going . . ."
>
> **—Meredith Scott, age 47**
> **7 years of TONE-UP**

stairs. Sleeping however, which is when your body does all its rebuilding and repairing, is considered aerobic because of all the constant energy it requires.

The time we burn the highest percentage of fat is about thirty minutes into an aerobic state. So, you may be thinking, "If I sleep eight hours and am burning the highest percentage of fat all night, why aren't I skinny?"

Well, the problem is that when you sleep or rest you burn only 1 per minute. (An active person burns more calories per minute because her metabolism is higher.) So half of that equals ½ calorie of fat burned per minute which equals only 240 calories of fat burned per eight hours of sleep. While doing a more active aerobic exercise for thirty minutes you can burn around eight calories per minute. Then you would utilize four calories of fat per minute which equals 120 calories of fat burned in just thirty minutes. Which seems like a better weight loss approach to you?

Let's not forget the most important reason for training, or exercising, our heart muscle both aerobically and anaerobically. It needs to be able to function at its full potential to prevent heart attacks, clogged arteries, and heart disease.

When I talk about aerobic exercise, I am referring to any activity which fulfills the these three factors recommended by the American College of Sports Medicine (ACSM): *Frequency, Duration, and Intensity.*

For *deconditioned people* (beginners), their recommendations are as follows:

1. **Frequency**, the number of times you work out in a week. Three days week is sufficient.
2. **Duration**, the number of minutes of aerobic exercise. Aerobic exercise must last from 20 to 60 minutes, exclusive of the warm up (the first 5 minutes to raise your heart rate) and the cool-down (the last 5 minutes to lower your heart rate.)
3. **Intensity**, the speed, or resistance you exercise with. To sufficiently burn fat, maintain your heart rate within your Target Heart Zone (explained below).

Aerobic (Cardiovascular Activities Include:

▶ Brisk (!) walking
▶ Running
▶ Cross-country skiing
▶ Aerobic stepping
▶ Skating
▶ Swimming

▶ Rope jumping
▶ Treadmill walking
▶ Aerobic dancing
▶ Stationary cycling
▶ Bicycling
▶ Stair climbing

According to the Fitness Resource Associates, "There is no best aerobic exercise other than the one that uses the large muscles of the body, encourages compliance, adheres to the above frequency, intensity, and duration guidelines and does so without providing undue physical stress or injury potential."

So, what does this all come down to?

1. **Find** a form of aerobic exercise that you enjoy.
2. **Warm up** by slowly and gently performing the activity that you have chosen to do.
3. **Raise** your pulse to your Target Heart Rate Zone (see below) while breathing regularly. Maintain it for 20 to 60 minutes.
4. **Cool down and stretch** appropriately.

To take your *heart rate*, turn one palm up. With your other hand, press all four fingers (not your thumb) gently on the radial (thumb) side of your arteries. Using a clock's second hand, count your heartbeats (starting with 1) for 10 seconds; then, multiply by 6 for a one minute count (Beats Per Minute).

Finding Your *TARGET HEART RATE ZONE*

First, you need to know your Resting Heart Rate (*RHR*). To get your *RHR*, take your pulse for three days first thing in the morning (before the alarm rings) and record it. Take the average of all three days.

The *Karvonen Formula* is used to calculate your Target Heart Rate Zone (**THRZ**) :
1. 220 minus your age,
2. minus your *RHR*,
3. multiplied by 60% and by 90%.
4. Add your *RHR* back onto both equations and you'll get your *THRZ*.

Sample—Melissa is 40 years old with a resting heart rate (*RHR*) of 60 beats per minute.

1. 220	2. 180	3. 120	120	4. 72	108
−40	−60	x .60	x .90	+60	+60
180	120	72	108	132	168

Therefore, Melissa's THRZ is 132-168 beats per minute.

"To maximize fat-burning: Exercise as hard as comfortably possible, for as long as possible, as often as possible."
—Dr. Daniel Kosich, Ph.D

Would the use of ankle or hand weights during my aerobic workout be beneficial?

Please do not use ankle or hand weights while participating in any aerobic activity. Combining the weights and the activity may be more detrimental than beneficial.

It drives me crazy when I see someone walking or running around my neighborhood with added weights on her wrists and/or ankles. Let me explain why.

When you swing your arms in their natural motion, your shoulders are working in a rather small range of motion. Adding weights will only make the muscles tighter in that particular movement pattern. If you increase the range of motion by making large swinging movements or circles, the weights add unnecessary stress to the shoulder girdle.

"Although I am not a fitness freak or extremely worried about having the perfect body, TONE-UP gave me the figure I always hoped to have.

Before I started TONE-UP, I was 30 pounds overweight, on a strict diet and doing high impact aerobics 5 to 6 days a week. I lost weight...up to a certain point.

My body refused to budge from a certain weight (unless I starved myself, which was never an option for a lady with an appetite like me!). I was thin, but flabby (loose skin!) and I was weak...this was not how I wanted to look or feel!

I started TONE-UP and soon looked ten pounds lighter simply by better posture and a tighter abdomen.

It's challenging but not impossible. It's up to you to go as far as you can go! TONE-UP is a work in progress no matter how long they've been doing it! It's a physical as well as mental challenge. I gained strength in every muscle in my body! But most important, besides an improved figure, was attaining a stronger spine and a stronger mind."

—*Melanie Uranitsch, Los Angeles, 29*
5 years of TONE-UP

Doing biceps curls while walking for twenty to sixty minutes not only overworks the front of the arm but can exaggerate a twisting movement in the mid back, and pressing the weights overhead puts a tremendous strain on the lower back.

When ankle weights are used while walking or running, they place added stress on your joints. Knees and hips are joints that already tend to wear down earlier than we'd like, so, why speed up the process?

If you are walking to lose weight there is such a marginal increase in energy expenditure when using light weights, it's not worth the effort and the risks.

So, *please, please, please*, keep the weights for your strength-training and lose the weights for your aerobic activities.

But, if you are dead set on adding weight in order to burn extra calories and you have no joint discomfort, I recommend wearing a weighted vest or belt. Placing the weight on the center of your body will allow your extremities more freedom and flexibility of movement.

Chapter 9

Just One Last Question

Why am I gaining weight if I'm exercising to lose it?
Initially you may gain a few pounds, because muscle weighs more than fat. Don't get discouraged. Don't become obsessed with what the scale says—it has way too much influence on our emotions. When you get off the scale you feel either elated or depressed. Who needs it?

You are reshaping your body and replacing fat with muscle. Fat occupies three times the amount of space that muscle does, so for every pound of fat you lose, you can gain three pounds of muscle and not add a dress size.

Go by how you look and feel. The mirror, measurements, "before" photos and body fat testing are better indices of how you are progressing. The best way to judge, however, is to ask yourself a few questions: How am I feeling? How do my clothes fit? Is my body becoming more toned and fit?

What is the best time of day to exercise?
Simply for routine sake, it's best to work out the same time each day, if possible. I recommend first thing in the day, because we tend to find excuses later. But any time will do.

Is it O.K. to eat before I do TONE-UP?

Yes. If you haven't eaten anything for a few hours, I suggest a piece of fresh fruit, vegetable, or a little protein before you work out. If you must eat a complete meal before exercising, make it very light, preferably vegetables, then give yourself at least sixty minutes to begin digesting it.

You need energy in order to sustain this workout. If you exercise on an empty stomach, you may get light-headed or nauseous. TONE-UP is a continuous workout that raises your heart rate and uses both your immediate and stored energy sources: sugar and fat. You use more energy than you think and if there's none available, you may not feel so well.

After exercising, wait an hour or so before eating, then make it a balanced, healthy snack or meal.

Will I get stomach cramps if I drink water while I exercise?

No. You need to stay hydrated. Drink water continuously a little at a time. Don't wait until you are thirsty. By then you are already dehydrated.

Dehydration can cause muscle cramping and fatigue, headaches and nausea.

Can leg exercises get rid of cellulite?

No. Cellulite is just a fancy name for fat and you cannot spot-reduce fat on legs by leg lifts alone.

Eating right plus habitual exercise can change that. When you lose fat, you lose it equally all over your body. Some areas may have a greater concentration of fat cells to begin with and therefore will appear to be the last place you lose it. But don't get discouraged—the shape and muscle tone of your legs will improve with the TONE-UP system.

The older I get, the more my body looks like my mother's! Is there anything I can do to prevent this?

Yes and no. Let me explain.

Yes. Be more active than your mother. Get in shape! Don't have the same lifestyle habits your mother had.

And no. Genetics plays a big part in your body type and shape. If your mother is an *apple shape*, bigger in the torso than the legs, and you tend to carry weight in your stomach too, that will be the last area of your body to lose fat. If you and she are *pear shapes*, you store more fat in your hips and thighs than the torso.

No matter where we store fat, we wish it were somewhere else, like maybe on someone else's body. Most women tend to have a heavier lower body than upper body. The good news is that it's healthier than the alternative because upper-body fat can accumulate around your heart and internal organs. The bad news is that lower-body fat is harder to lose.

But remember that while no amount of exercise is going to change your inherent design, you can certainly reshape your form by exercising and eating right.

I was skinny as a child but started gaining weight at thirty-five. Am I destined to get fatter and fatter?

No. We are born with a predetermined number of fat cells decided by genetics. After that, there are three more times in a woman's life when we can increase that amount: during infancy, puberty, and pregnancy.

If you are not genetically determined to be fat, you start off with fewer fat cells than someone who is genetically a fat person. If you gain a lot of weight during any of the above-mentioned times of your life, then you will accumulate more fat cells.

51

When you gain weight, the fat cells fill up, and when you lose weight, they empty out. Obviously, the more fat cells you have, the fatter you can become. So, if you were always been heavy as a child and growing up, it will be more difficult, but not impossible, for you to become a thin person, and vise versa.

Therefore, to answer the question: *No*, if you didn't gain weight until you were thirty-five, you will probably not become fatter and fatter unless you radically change your lifestyle and eating habits.

What is most important, though, is to lead the healthiest, most active lifestyle you can, and make the best of what you've got, because genetics determines only part of our destiny and we determine the rest.

Should I exercise if I don't feel well?

A doctor friend of mine once put it to me in very simple terms:

If you are sick above the neck, e.g., a cold or headache, yes, it's probably fine to exercise. If you are sick below the neck, e.g., sore throat, chest pains, cough, fever, stomach problems, no. Use your good sense, especially if you may infect others.

If I have arthritis, osteoporosis, fibromyalgia, or a "bad" joint is TONE-UP dangerous for me?

No. When prescribed by your doctor, exercise is excellent for easing painful joints and increasing bone density. According to Dr. Neil Gordon of the Cooper Institute for Aerobic Research in Dallas, "The four-letter word people with arthritis must avoid using is 'quit.' Many people with arthritis can maintain flexibility, or restore it, through a well-designed exercise program that is implemented gradually and regularly."

Osteoporosis, the thinning of bones, is a major cause of disability among older women. It has been called a silent disease, since you may not be aware you have it until you fracture a bone. Although it may not become a problem until menopause, lifelong habits are the best prevention. In fact, your activity level as an adolescent has a crucial effect on your chances of getting osteoporosis as an adult.

From my experience, when someone says she has a *bad* something, the pain is usually caused by weak or unbalanced muscles surrounding the joints that hurt. If that's the case, the TONE-UP system is exactly what you need.

If I'm so sore that I can barely move, should I work out again or wait until I'm no longer sore?

First evaluate your soreness. Is it muscular, like a charley horse, or is it in your joints, for example, knees, lower back? If it's an achy nonspecific feeling, yes, you should work out again. If it's an injury, you need to reconsider.

Soreness means that you've overworked unused muscles, and/or perhaps you didn't stretch to your ability. I think of this as *muscle awareness*. Performing the same exercise at a slightly lower intensity will help work out the tenderness. If you don't work the soreness out, the next time you exercise you will be essentially starting over again, and the same thing may happen.

There are two types of injuries: acute and chronic. An acute injury is one that happens suddenly, like a sprain or a break. A chronic injury is one that is marked by long duration or frequent recurrence, like tennis elbow or carpal tunnel syndrome.

If you have any injury, make sure you get advice from your doctor before starting an exercise program.

If you feel as if you pulled or strained a muscle, sports doctors recommend you apply the R.I.C.E. therapy. That stands for *Rest, Ice, Compression, Elevation.* For the first 48 hours after an injury, apply ice every few hours for 20 minutes. After that initial period, you may alternate ice and moist heat, but always end with ice. Apply as often as needed.

If your aches are in your joints you should either reconsider the exercises you're doing, pay extra attention to the details of how to execute them, cut back on repetitions or weight, or modify them to fit your particular needs.

In any case, listen to your body: let the tender areas rest for a couple of days until the soreness goes away, but continue moderately with the rest of your program.

Chapter 10

Six Points You Need to Know

A. Your Workout Space & Attire

B. Muscle Balancing

C. Torso Stabilization & Neutral Alignment

D. Kinesiology & Kinesthetic Awareness

E. About Abdominals

F. Warming-Up & Stretching

A. Your Workout Space & Attire

Setting up your own space is important. Make sure it is far from any distractions. This is what I recommend:

- A small, well ventilated area in which to lie down and stand. You need to be able to put your arms in all directions and not hit anything
- A comfortable exercise mat to lie on
- A chair without arms (e.g., a folding chair)
- A set of light hand-held weights
     A "set" is two weights
     Beginner: 2 or 3 lb.
     Intermediate: 4 or 5 lb.
- Lightweight, nonrestrictive clothing
- Bare feet* or <u>flexible</u> sneakers, if you must
- A mirror to check body positioning; to be used only objectively
- This book and/or audio tape
- A camera to take your "before" photos now; also to be used objectively
- Plenty of water to drink

* I recommend bare feet so you can build strength and mobility in *all* your muscles and joints. Look at your favorite old shoes. You'll see how all your bad habits and alignment problems manifest themselves in the way you've worn them out. Save the tennis shoes for tennis and join me *sans shoes*.

B. Muscle Balancing

Have you ever noticed after you sit at a computer all day, how good it feels to stand up and place your hands on your lower back and arch slightly? Or after a long night's sleep, how soothing it feels to reach all the way up?

Ever had a major calf cramp in the middle of the night?

Have you ever noticed how large the thighs of speed skaters are? The overly developed lower bodies of bicycle racers with their lesser developed upper bodies? How amateur bodybuilders tend to have round shoulders and arms they can't straighten?

All of the above are examples of muscle imbalances.

When you sit at a desk all day, your chest muscles, shoulders, and the front of your hips get shortened and tightened. Sleeping in a fetal position causes your feet to point, which can ultimately contract your calves so much that they cramp.

> "I consider TONE-UP my antidote to the stress of my work. My back has never felt better. My posture is great, even at the computer. I think of the work that I do during her class as an investment in my own present and future health.
>
> I recommend Suesan's methods to anyone thinking 'there's got to be more to life than feeling like a weakling'!"
>
> —*Linda Havlik, age 49*
> *4 years of TONE-UP*

Athletes who are single-sport specific tend to get overly developed in the muscles primarily used. The results may be ideal for competition, but they are neither functionally correct nor aesthetically pleasing.

You know how important "how many" and "how heavy" are when referring to bench presses and biceps curls. Amateur bodybuilders tend to concentrate more on the chest and biceps than the back and triceps which causes the round shouldered and bent elbow stereotypical bodybuilder physique.

> "TONE-UP is excellent for correcting postural problems. Suesan's exercises are based on perfect physiological balance. It's the best overall structural toning I've ever seen, and there's no stress to the knees or spinal joints."
> —*Dr. Deborah Holtzman, age 34*
> *Doctor of Chiropractic,*
> *1 year of TONE-UP*

We are made up of opposing muscles that are directly opposite each other.

Our major opposing muscle groups are:

quadriceps (thigh) vs. *hamstrings* (back of thigh),

adductors (inner thigh) vs. *abductors* (outer thigh),

gastrocnemius and *soleus* (calf) vs. *tibialis anterior* (shin),

iliopsoas (front of pelvis) vs. *gluteals* (buttocks),

biceps (front of upper arm) vs. *triceps* (back of upper arm),

pectorals (chest) vs. *trapezius* and *rhomboids* (mid-back),

rectus abdominis and *obliques* (abdomen) vs. *erector spinae* (lower back),

deltoids (shoulders) vs. *latissimus dorsi* (sides of back).

When worked unevenly, you can cause an imbalance.

The activities you do every day greatly affect the structure of your body. The way you walk, stand, sit, lie, and drive your car make an impact on your posture and presentation.

Muscle balancing is very important. While doing the TONE-UP system, make sure you do *all* the exercises and not just the ones you like or think you need.

C. Torso Stabilization & Neutral Alignment

Torso Stabilization is a posture, balance, and alignment awareness that I will remind you of while exercising. It applies to all my exercises.

The most important part of your body is your torso, or your center. You can exist without extremities, but not without a torso.

Whether you are exercising or vacuuming your rug, you need to have supportive strength in the center of your body. You need to have complete consciousness and control of what your body is doing while performing any exercise or task. Without that awareness and control you are setting yourself up for injuries and accidents.

For example: While doing *Biceps Curls*, keep your shoulders and upper arms from moving and your abdomen contracted to keep your back from moving. The only part of you that moves to execute a *Biceps Curl* is your forearm.

Neutral Alignment is perfect posture, as described on the following page. When I refer to neutral alignment, the positioning is relative to the rest of your body, not to the direction you are facing in the room. Whether you are standing up, lying on the floor, or standing on your head (which we won't), your *neutral alignment* always remains the same.

Neutral Alignment Cues and Reminders

Imagine you are suspended from the ceiling by a string attached to the highest part of your head, which is right above your spine.

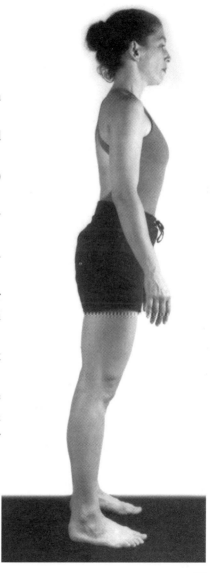

- Focus straight ahead
- Back of neck lengthened
- Chin slightly down
- Shoulders pressed down away from your ears
- Shoulder blades pulled down and gently back
- Center of chest (sternum) open and lifted
- Abdominals (and belly button) lifted and tight
- Front of pelvis flat; buttocks relaxed
- A natural curve in lumbar (lower) spine (not tipped under)
- Knees extended, but not locked
- Weight primarily on the balls of your feet, with your heels on floor for balance.

D. Kinesiology & Kinesthetic Awareness

Kinesiology is the study of the principles of human movement. Here are some basic principles.

Primary Mover is the main muscle group you are working. For example, your chest (pectoralis) is the primary mover in a *Push-up*.

Secondary Movers are the assisting muscles. The back of your arms (triceps) are the secondary movers in a *Push-up*.

Stabilizers are the muscles that hold the rest of your body in place so you can perform the exercise correctly. The back (latissimus dorsi) and shoulders (deltoids) are the stabilizers in a *Push-up*.

Kinesthetic Awareness is the ability to know exactly where and how your body is placed without having to check in a mirror. For example, if you don't hit yourself in the head during *Triceps Overhead* (pg. 98), your kinesthetic awareness is pretty good!

Once you become physically conscious of your body's neutral alignment and torso stabilization, you will develop your kinesthetic awareness. You will become able to readjust yourself to a more attractive and healthier body alignment in your habitual postures.

E. About Abdominals

The rectus abdominis and the obliques are the muscles of the abdominal group that are primarily used to move the torso. They connect the ribcage to the pelvis. The main purposes of your abdominal muscles are to turn you side to side, bend you forward from the waist, aid your posture, and hold in your internal organs.

I believe the main purpose of doing *Sit-ups* is so you can sit up, get up, and stay up without having to roll over, push yourself up, or stabilize yourself with your arms.

During the normal course of a day you need to use your abdominal muscles almost constantly for reaching, standing, turning, leaning, and even laughing. These endurance muscles will not develop into bulging muscles, like your thighs or shoulders. They are designed to work nonstop for long periods of time and can ultimately form smooth, almost flat abdominals.

Will you ever get a flat stomach? The abdominal wall is a slightly rounded muscle to begin with, and as women, we have to pack quite a few internal organs inside a small space. The area below your belly button may always tend to stick out a bit no matter what you do. Plus, we tend to store fat on our abdomen for childbearing.

Could you ever get that six-pack cut abdominal look? Well, it depends. That look is achieved by having a developed abdominal wall plus minimal fat on top of it. Our muscle fibers have three sets of ridges, called tendinous inscriptions, and if there is absolutely no fat between the skin and muscle, you get that appearance.

63

How do you figure out whether your abdomen is mostly fat or muscle? Lie on your back with your knees bent and feet flat on the floor. Crunch up, or lift your head and upper back off the floor, so your abdominal muscles get tight. Can you feel where your abdomen is relatively hard? That's the muscle. Anything that you can grab with your hand is the fat. *Sit-ups* will tighten the muscle but won't get rid of that extra stuff on top.

No exercise can "spot-reduce" a specific area. *Sit-ups* will tighten and strengthen your abdominal muscles, which in turn eases the burden your lower back is carrying. Your posture will improve, your lower back pain will disappear, your waist will become tighter, your stomach will become flatter, and anything that's on top of it will look better.

Have you ever had a well-defined flat stomach? Are you a man? Under 21? If you answered *no* to any of these questions, then you may never achieve "the look." But is that really so important? Do we need to look like we have the stomach of an adolescent boy?

If your abdomen is weak, your back muscles (the opposing muscles) have to do most of the work, and therefore get tired. That's why so many people believe they have a "bad back." In actuality, their back muscles are stronger than their abdominals and just can't handle the load any more.

While training your abdominal muscles you should do two things. Alternate between:
1. Working continually as long as possible to build endurance, and
2. Holding your abdomen in a contracted position to build strength.

Abdominals need to be trained not to quit on you when you really need them.

Fortunately, these muscles recover very quickly, so when they get tired you just need a short break before you can start up again. Quick recovery also means you can do abdominal exercises as often as you want!

While performing my *Sit-ups (Abdominal Work)*, concentrate carefully on proper form and technique, and on torso stabilization and isolation. You move only the ribs and/or the pelvis. Everything else just comes along for the ride.

Your chest stays in an open neutral position. Your head maintains one comfortable position the whole time so you don't start "nodding," which puts strain on your neck. And your arms and legs are used simply for intensity and variety.

"We like the way Suesan challenges us—bring us right up to the edge of what we are capable of. This class really builds confidence as well as muscle strength and balance. We further appreciate the way Suesan very thoroughly explains the physiological connections and benefits deriving from each exercise."

—*Inge and Walter Knapp,*
senior citizens
7 months of TONE-UP

F. Warming-Up & Stretching

"What's the difference between warming up and stretching? Do I really need to do them both?"

Warming up and stretching are equally important and completely different.

Warming up can be as simple as a lower-intensity simulation of the exercise you'll be doing soon at a higher-intensity, for example, walking before you run. A proper warm up will prepare your body for what's to come so you won't get injured. It is done prior to activity.

Static stretching is a sustained, long, duration hold of an already warmed-up muscle that is designed to increase length and flexibility and reduce stiffness. After your warm up, after you work a specific muscle group, and at the end of your activity are the optimal times for static stretches.

If you bounce in a stretch, your body reacts with a stretch reflex in which your muscles tighten up to protect themselves from injury, which makes the stretch counterproductive.

Instead of bouncing, concentrate on elongating and relaxing your muscles. Take a deep breath so you can exhale as you relax into each stretch for 20 to 60 seconds. Move slowly and smoothly from one stretch to another. Each time you do a static stretch, attempt to increase your flexibility a little more than the previous time.

Chapter 11

The Tone-Up™ System

The following pages of photographs represent form and function of each exercise, not variations and repetitions. Each exercise, when done properly and to the point at which you feel the muscles working, will yield great results.

Begin by performing at least 20 repetitions of each exercise, and increase the number as your strength improves. Please pay careful attention and take all instructions personally.

If you feel you need a little extra motivation or push, consider purchasing the *Be Your Best Body*™, 60-minute Tone-Up™ Workout Audiocassette Tape, which is sold separately and was designed in conjunction with this book. Each exercise demonstrated in the book is taught, by me, in detail, on the cassette. It's just like I'm right there with you in an authentic Tone-Up™ class.

If you feel light-headed during your workout, walk around the room or sit with your head held lower than your heart. While exercising, your blood pumps to the muscles you're working. Occasionally, if you stop suddenly there may not be enough time for the blood to flow back to your head. This causes the blood to pool in your extremities which may make you feel light-headed or nauseous. There is a greater tendency for this to happen if you haven't eaten for a while, are out of shape, or have very low blood pressure.

If that's the case, take a short rest until you're ready to resume.

OK—here we go! Just remember —TONE-UP™ is meant to be challenging, not impossible!

The basic TONE-UP system, as demonstrated in *Be Your Best Body*, is also available on a 60-minute audio cassette tape which was designed specifically to go with this book.

This TONE-UP class is taught by Suesan in its actual class format and is set to original soft jazz music that everyone will enjoy.

So, order today so you can receive the best results in the least amount of time.

You may purchase the workout tape, plus additional books and tapes for your friends and family, by either mailing a coupon from the back of this book to Tone-Up Publishing, P.O. Box 30058, Santa Barbara, Ca. 93130, or emailing us at ToneUpPub@aol.com.

Part A

Warm-Up and Legs

Walking in Place
(warms up feet, ankles, and calves)
1. Begin by standing. Place your hands on the back of a chair, kitchen counter, or barre. Feet slightly behind you. Keep the balls of your feet on the floor and roll each heel, one at a time, down to the floor.

Calf Raises
2. Start with both feet flat on the floor. Keep legs straight and pelvis pressed slightly forward.

2a. Use your full range of motion as you roll your heels up and down.

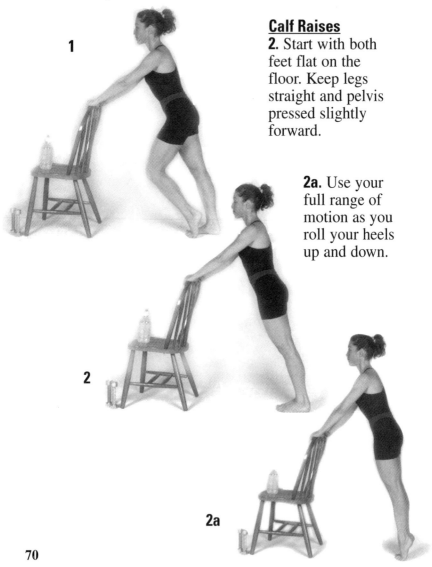

1

2

2a

70

Single Leg Calf Raises
3. Wrap one foot around the other ankle.
3a. Roll heel up and down. If it's too difficult, repeat both legs together again.

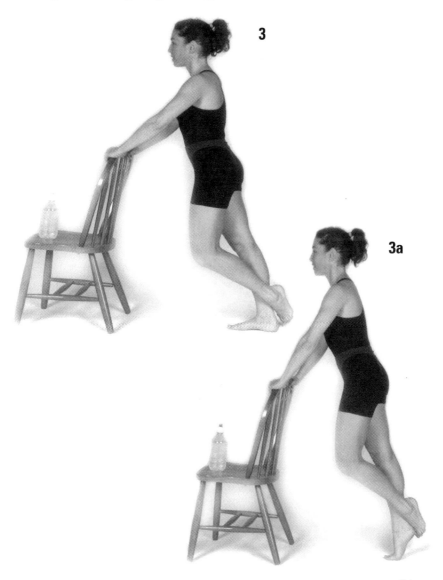

3

3a

Toe Taps
(shins)

4. Place one foot forward and one foot back. With forward knee bent and rear knee straight, tap your forward foot. Keep your hips stable.

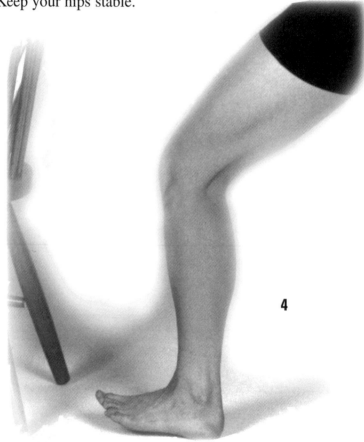

4

Ankle Circles
(not pictured)

This is a stretch to relax your ankle muscles after you finish the *Toe Taps* (#4), Place your forward foot behind you with your knees close together. Inscribe a large circle with your big toe to circle your ankle.

Repeat *Toe Taps and Ankle Circles* with other leg.

Plie (plee-yay) *a ballet term meaning bending of knees with your back straight*

Plies in First Position

6. Place one hand on the back of a chair and the other arm out to the side. Begin with your legs straight, turned out from the top of the thigh, and heels together. Upper body remains in neutral alignment. Keep your weight primarily on your heels, toes relaxed.

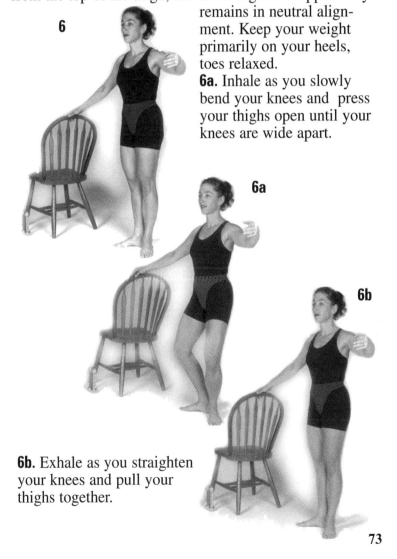

6a. Inhale as you slowly bend your knees and press your thighs open until your knees are wide apart.

6b. Exhale as you straighten your knees and pull your thighs together.

Heel Lifts

7. In *First Position Plie*, roll up onto your toes. Press your thighs out and your heels forward. Keep your weight primarily toward your bigger toes.
7a. When you roll your heels down, press them into the floor. Repeat.

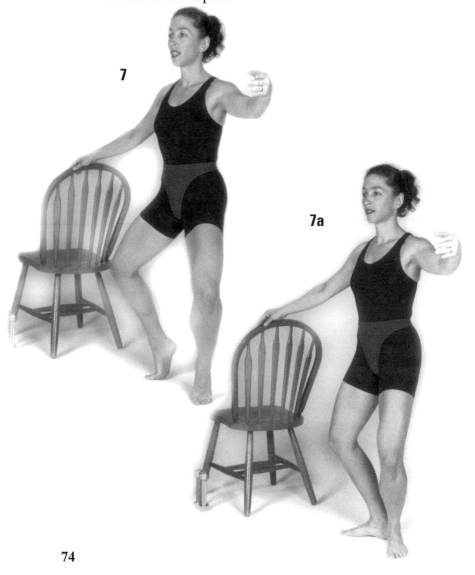

74

Plie Presses

Remain in *First Position Plie* with heels lifted.
There are two parts to this exercise.

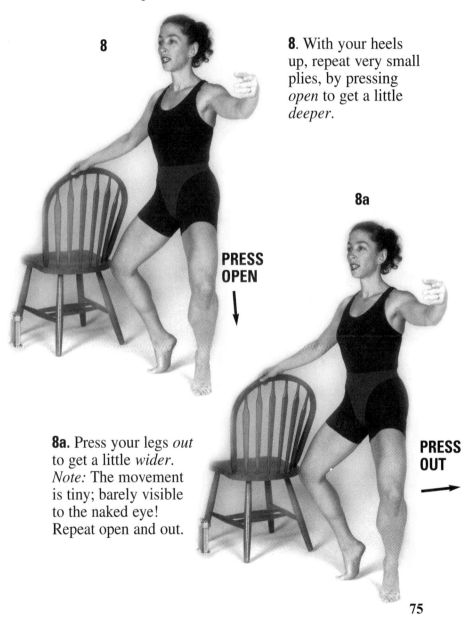

8

8. With your heels
up, repeat very small
plies, by pressing
open to get a little
deeper.

8a

**PRESS
OPEN**

↓

8a. Press your legs *out*
to get a little *wider.*
Note: The movement
is tiny; barely visible
to the naked eye!
Repeat open and out.

**PRESS
OUT**

→

75

Deep Plies

9. While in *First Position Plie*, with your heels lifted, inhale as you slowly press your thighs out as wide as you can, so your body lowers into a deep plie.
Keep your shoulders directly over your hips, and your hips over your heels.

9

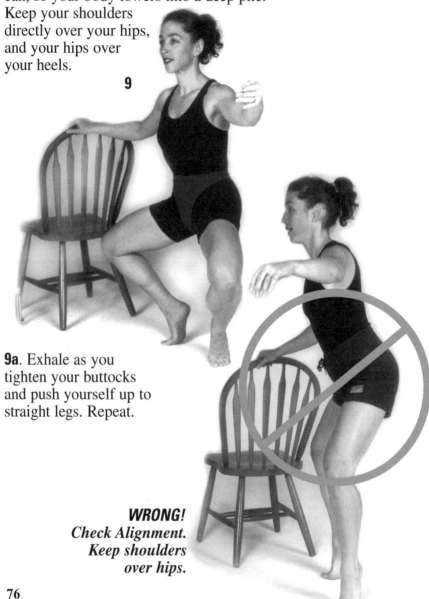

9a. Exhale as you tighten your buttocks and push yourself up to straight legs. Repeat.

WRONG!
Check Alignment.
Keep shoulders
over hips.

Balance

10. A balance is a held position, which could be any position. A *balance* should feel comfortable. When you are balanced, or "centered," it will feel effortless. When you are comfortably balanced, you are either in perfect alignment or just very lucky! You need to concentrate primarily on stabilizing your torso.

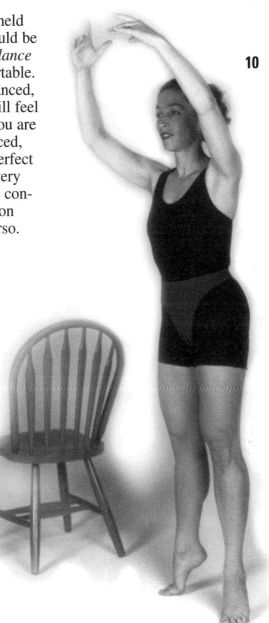

10

Plies in a Wide Second Position

11. Stand with your feet wider apart than hip width, your weight primarily on your heels, your toes relaxed.

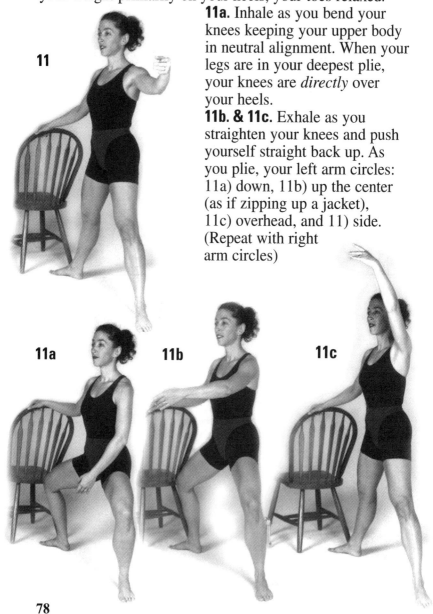

11a. Inhale as you bend your knees keeping your upper body in neutral alignment. When your legs are in your deepest plie, your knees are *directly* over your heels.

11b. & 11c. Exhale as you straighten your knees and push yourself straight back up. As you plie, your left arm circles: 11a) down, 11b) up the center (as if zipping up a jacket), 11c) overhead, and 11) side. (Repeat with right arm circles)

78

Wide Second Position Plie Presses

12. While in a deep *Wide Second Position Plie* you perform the plie presses open and out, and repeat. (See exercise #8 on page 75).

12

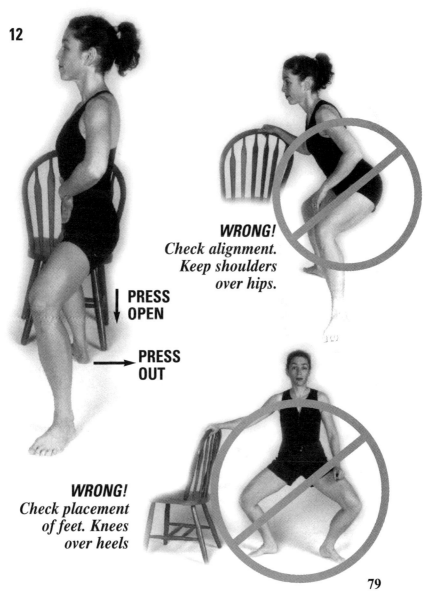

PRESS
OPEN

PRESS
OUT

WRONG!
Check alignment.
Keep shoulders
over hips.

WRONG!
Check placement
of feet. Knees
over heels

79

Turn the Leg In and Out (hip rotation)
In a *deep Wide Second Position Plie*:
13. *LIFT* one heel up and down, then keep heel lifted and perform small plies,
13a. *ROTATE* that leg *in* from the hip so your knee points down, pulse your knee down toward the floor,

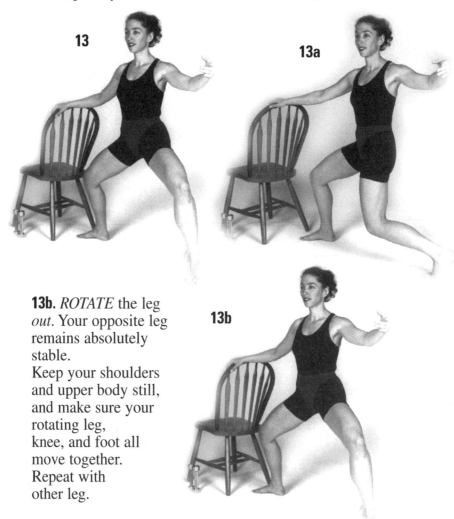

13.

13a.

13b. *ROTATE* the leg *out*. Your opposite leg remains absolutely stable.
Keep your shoulders and upper body still, and make sure your rotating leg, knee, and foot all move together. Repeat with other leg.

13b

Part B

Lunges

Stationary Lunges

Start by standing with your legs parallel (toes pointing straight ahead), facing and holding the back of a chair.
14. Place one foot directly below and parallel to your hands, and place the other leg far enough behind you that the heel can't possibly touch the floor. Your weight is distributed evenly between your forward foot and the ball of your rear foot.

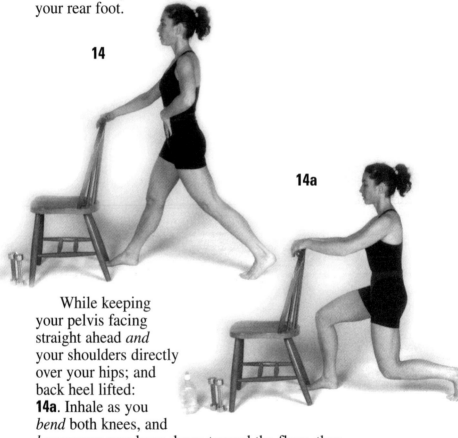

14

14a

While keeping your pelvis facing straight ahead *and* your shoulders directly over your hips; and back heel lifted:
14a. Inhale as you *bend* both knees, and *lower* your rear knee down toward the floor, then
14. exhale as you *straighten* both legs at the same time back to the beginning lunge position. Repeat.
Repeat with other leg.

Back Lunges

I also refer to these as *Regular Lunges*. This lunge works your forward leg. The rear leg is for balance, not support. The action of lowering and raising your whole body with your forward leg works the buttocks and the hamstring muscles. Follow these directions extra carefully! To get good results, they must be done with your best form. Remember to keep your torso stabilized.

15. Start (and finish) by standing with your hands on the back of a chair and your feet together in parallel position (toes pointing straight ahead).

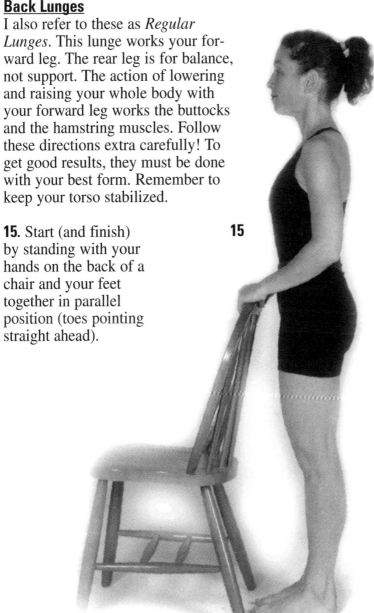

15

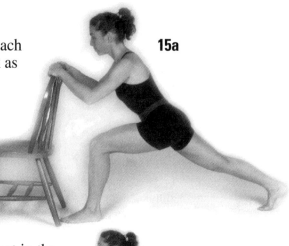

15a

15a. Inhale as you reach one straight leg back as far as possible.

As you do, make sure that:

1. Your hands stay on the chair
2. With each repetition, you place your foot in the exact same spot
3. Your body weight is primarily on your forward heel
4. Your forward knee stays directly over the heel with your leg bent at a 90% angle
5. Your forward ankle and shin remain stable
6. The rear heel remains lifted
7. Top of your head goes close to the chair
8. Your shoulders stay directly over your forward leg.

15b

15b. Exhale as you press down with forward heel and push straight back up to standing. Repeat with other leg.

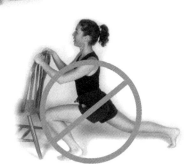

WRONG!
Check alignment

16. HAMSTRING STRETCH

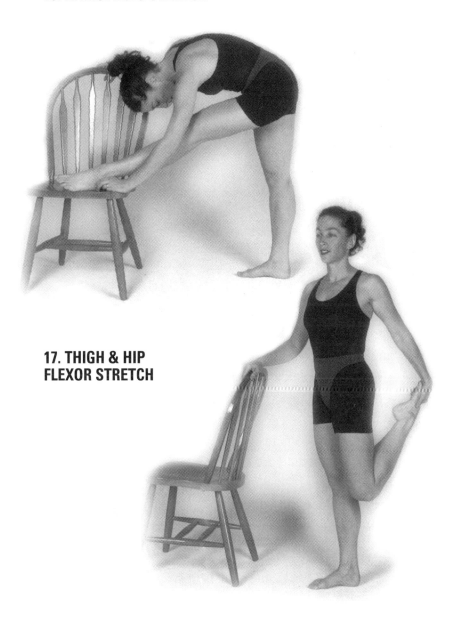

17. THIGH & HIP
FLEXOR STRETCH

Part C

Additional Stretches
(not on audio tape)

BACK "CAT" STRETCH

Start with your feet hip-width apart, toes facing straight ahead, and knees bent.

Place your hands on your thighs and *round* your back by tucking your pelvis under, placing your chin to your chest, and looking at your (concave) abdomen. Then, *flatten* your back by pushing your hips all the way back. Round your back again, bend your knees a little more, tuck pelvis under deeper and hold the stretch for 30 seconds.

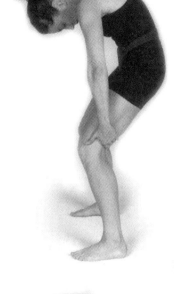

ROTATING BACK STRETCH

Flatten your back again, move your feet wider apart into a *Wide Second Position Plie*. Press your hands on your inner thighs for support and sit all the way back. You are now in a *turned-out squat position*. Press your left hand against left thigh and turn right, directly around your spine. Repeat to other side.

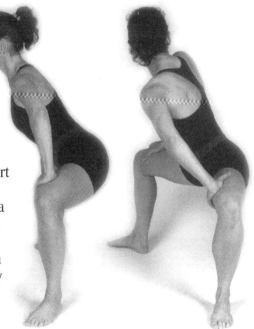

INNER THIGH AND HAMSTRING STRETCHES

Remain in the turned-out squat position (see above) and place your elbows against your thighs. Keep your weight on your heels and sit way back.

Without letting your hips drop down, press your thighs out as wide as you can. Your upper body will counterbalance your lower body. Hold the stretch for 20 to 30 seconds. This position is not for comfort, it's for a deep stretch!

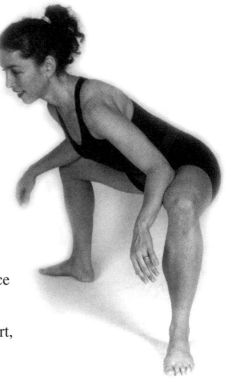

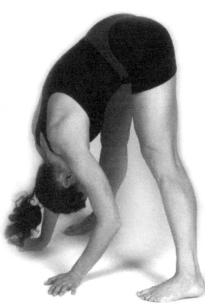

When you've had enough, slowly turn your legs back into parallel position, straighten your legs, and hang your head toward the floor. Bend your knees slightly and roll up slowly, one vertebra at a time, until you're standing fully erect in perfect alignment.

Back, Biceps & Shoulders

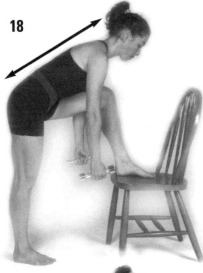

18

Back Rows
(with weights)

18. Begin with one foot placed on a chair and other leg straight. Bend forward from your hips, push your hips back and keep your head in line with your spine. With the weights in your hands, hang your arms straight down with your knuckles facing in.

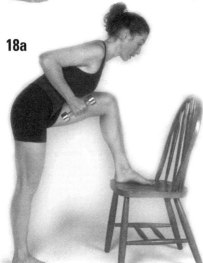

18a

18a. First inhale, then exhale as you bend your elbows and lift your hands to your ribcage. Squeeze your shoulder blades and elbows toward each other as you open your chest.

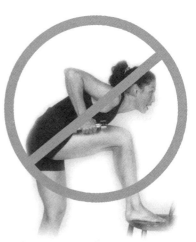

WRONG!
Straighten
back & align
neck.

19

Back Flyes
(with weights)
19. Same position as for
Back Rows (see above).
Keep elbows slightly bent.
19a. Inhale, then exhale as
you slowly open your arms
wide, and lift side as high
as you can. Keep your
shoulders pulled down, and
squeeze your shoulder
blades toward each other.

19a

Inhale as you
release your
arms down.
Keep your torso
stabilized. Move
only from your
shoulders.
Both exercises, the
Rows and the
Flyes, work the
muscles up the
center and the sides
of your back. Torso
stabilized!

91

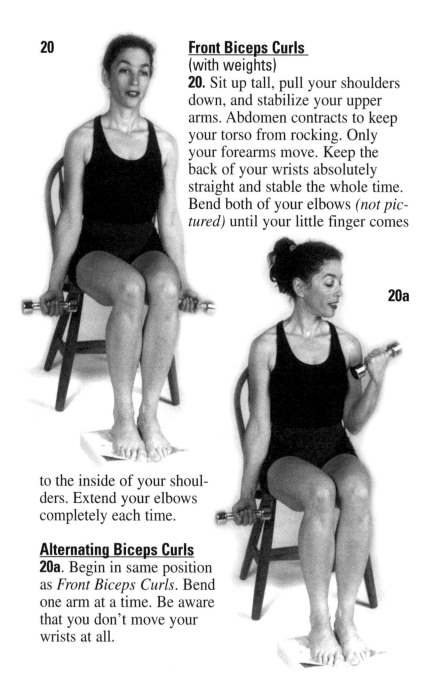

20

Front Biceps Curls
(with weights)
20. Sit up tall, pull your shoulders down, and stabilize your upper arms. Abdomen contracts to keep your torso from rocking. Only your forearms move. Keep the back of your wrists absolutely straight and stable the whole time. Bend both of your elbows *(not pictured)* until your little finger comes

20a

to the inside of your shoulders. Extend your elbows completely each time.

Alternating Biceps Curls
20a. Begin in same position as *Front Biceps Curls*. Bend one arm at a time. Be aware that you don't move your wrists at all.

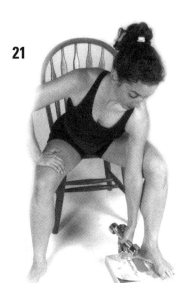

21

One Arm Bicep Curls
(with both weights in one hand)
Start sitting in a chair, feet wide apart.
To get into the correct position:
21. Lean forward from your hips with your back flat. (If you find you have to bend over very far, place your right foot on a phone book for added height.)
Reach your right hand (holding both weights) towards the floor. Rest that arm against your right leg for support. Turn your upper body slightly towards your left leg.

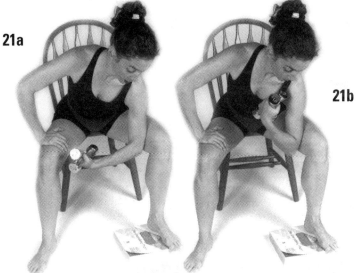

21a

21b

21a. & 21b. With your palm up, curl your right hand across the front of your torso, and up to the right shoulder while keeping it close to your body. Keep your wrist absolutely stable the whole time. When you curl up, lead with your knuckles, and when you go down, lead with the back of your wrist.
Repeat with other arm.

93

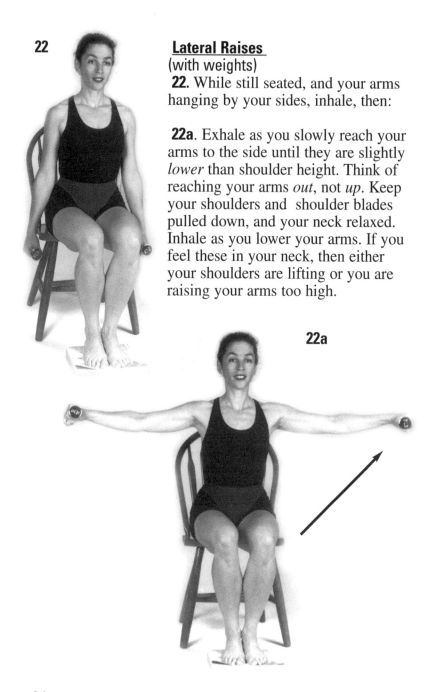

22

Lateral Raises
(with weights)

22. While still seated, and your arms hanging by your sides, inhale, then:

22a. Exhale as you slowly reach your arms to the side until they are slightly *lower* than shoulder height. Think of reaching your arms *out*, not *up*. Keep your shoulders and shoulder blades pulled down, and your neck relaxed. Inhale as you lower your arms. If you feel these in your neck, then either your shoulders are lifting or you are raising your arms too high.

22a

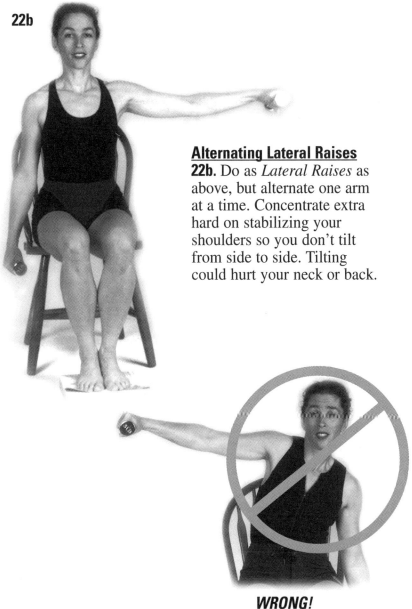

22b

Alternating Lateral Raises
22b. Do as *Lateral Raises* as above, but alternate one arm at a time. Concentrate extra hard on stabilizing your shoulders so you don't tilt from side to side. Tilting could hurt your neck or back.

WRONG!
Sit up tall & keep shoulders level.

95

Chest & Triceps

Push-Ups

23. Start by kneeling on your hands and knees. Place your hands directly in front of your shoulders. The placement of your knees is determined by your strength. The farther back you place your knees, the more body weight you will be pushing, therefore, the harder the *Push-ups* will be. During the entire *Push-up*, keep your shoulder blades wide apart, chest open, abdomen tight, and hips lifted slightly up.

23a. As you lower your body by bending your elbows, your chest leads (*not* your face), and **23b.** goes between your hands without "scrunching" your shoulder blades together.

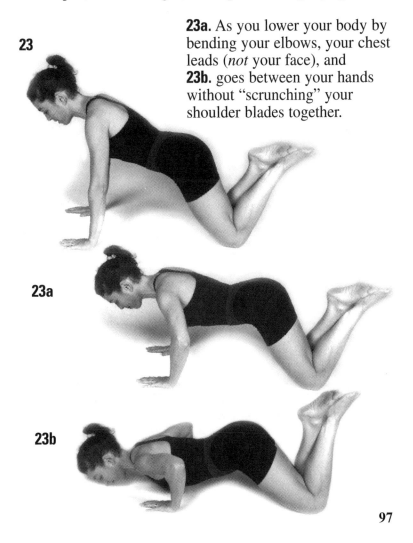

23

23a

23b

Triceps Overhead (with weights)
24. Lie on your back with your arms extended directly over your shoulders up toward the ceiling with your palms facing each other.

24a. Inhale as you bend your elbows until the weights touch the top of your shoulders. Exhale as you fully extend your arms again. Your upper arms remain stabilized so your elbows stay close together, and point straight to ceiling the whole time. As you bend and extend your elbows in a full range of motion, the weight will arc behind your ears. Keep your wrists straight so they don't "flick" at the top of the movement.

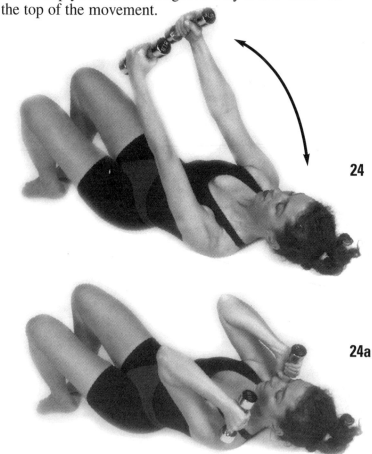

24

24a

90° Angle Tricep Presses (with weights)

25. Stay in the *Triceps Overhead* position as above. Bend your elbows into a 90° angle (forearms parallel with the floor). This is the starting and ending position. Imagine you are doing tiny *karate chops*, by moving your forearms up in a small range of motion (two inches) and back to ninety degrees.

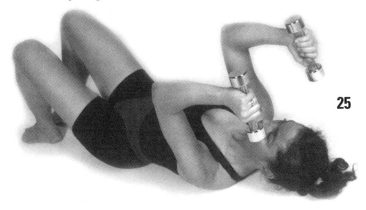

25

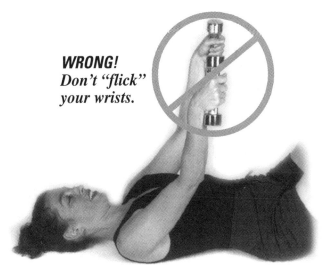

WRONG!
Don't "flick"
your wrists.

Shoulder, Chest & Biceps Stretch

26. Clasp your hands behind your back, open your chest and lift your chin slightly. Breathe and hold for 20 to 30 seconds.

26

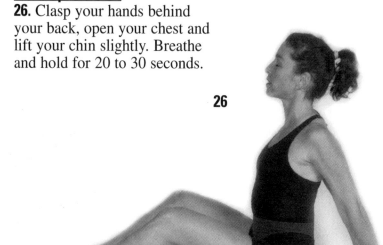

Triceps Stretch

27

27. Reach one arm overhead; bend the elbow and place that hand on the back of the same shoulder. With your other hand, push the elbow back gently. Breathe and hold stretch for 20 to 30 seconds. Repeat on the other side.

100

Part F

Abdominal Work
(Sit-Ups)

Half-Way Down Crunches
28. Sit straight up on the floor with you knees bent and your feet flat on the floor. Hold lightly onto the back of your thighs.

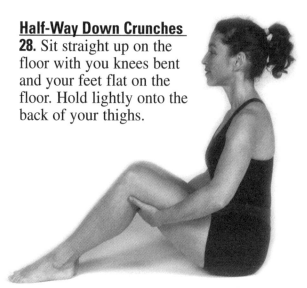

28

28a. Round your back until you are halfway down to the floor. While you stay in the deep pelvic tilt, keep your shoulders and neck relaxed and concentrate on your abdomen.

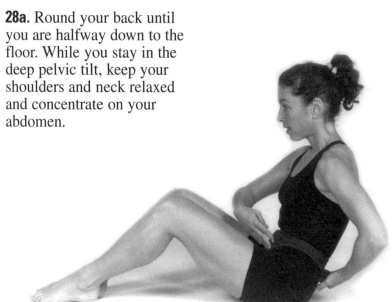

28a
"Tuck your pelvis under"

28b. and 28c. Contract (tighten & shorten) your abdomen by pressing (or bowing) your ribcage down towards your pelvis. The only part of you that moves is your ribcage. The range of motion is small. Keep your pelvis and legs absolutely still. Repeat the exercise by contracting and releasing your abdominal muscles.

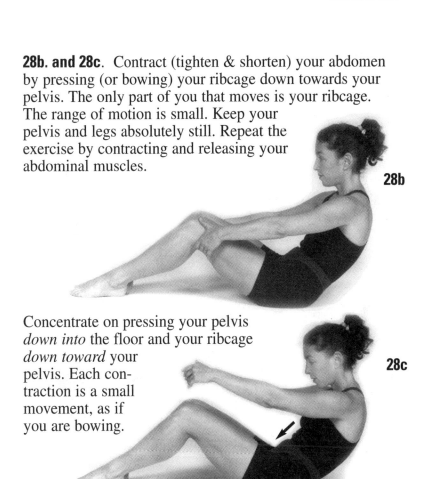

28b

Concentrate on pressing your pelvis *down into* the floor and your ribcage *down toward* your pelvis. Each contraction is a small movement, as if you are bowing.

28c

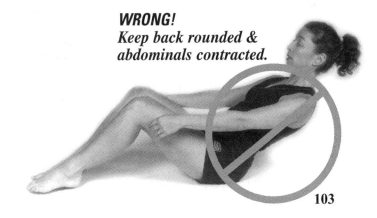

WRONG!
Keep back rounded &
abdominals contracted.

103

Half-Way-Down Turns

29. Stay in the deep pelvic tilt. Either keep your hands by your knees or hold lightly behind your thighs. Imagine your body is intersected down the middle. Don't cross the mid-line; just pivot around it, as if pivoting around a pole.

29

29a. & 29b. Focus straight ahead, keep your spine centered and rounded, and turn your ribcage side to side. Don't let your hips or legs move. If you feel these in the front

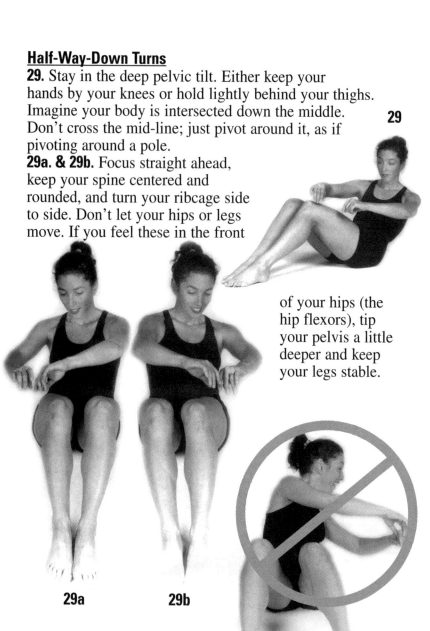

of your hips (the hip flexors), tip your pelvis a little deeper and keep your legs stable.

29a   **29b**

WRONG!
Don't turn so far.

Oblique Crunches

30. Lie on your back with one leg up toward the ceiling, and one foot on the floor. To get into the correct starting position: Hold onto the back on one leg and lift your shoulder blades (back bones) completely off the floor. Your body weight should be 99% on your pelvis and 1% on your lower foot. Next, support the crown (top) of your head with your hand. Then, rotate your upper body from the waist so your chest, elbow, and nose are all facing your lifted leg. "Nail" your opposite hip into the floor. Inhale, then exhale as you contract (tighten, shorten, and bow) and release toward your lifted leg.

30

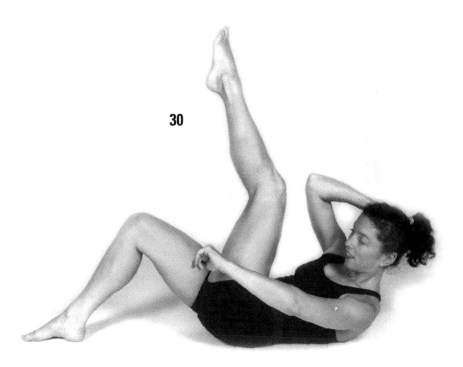

Legs-Up Crunches

31. Remain on the floor and raise both legs up towards the ceiling. Again, place most of your body weight on your pelvis. Lift your shoulder blades completely off the floor so your back in rounded. Use both hands to support the crown of your head, and point your elbows toward your legs. (If you cannot keep your shoulder blades off the floor, use one hand to hold onto the back of your leg to keep your upper body lifted.) Keep your chest open, your chin a few inches from your chest, and your jaw relaxed. Don't pull on your head. Let it rest in your hands. Then, exhale as you perform the "crunches" (or contractions).

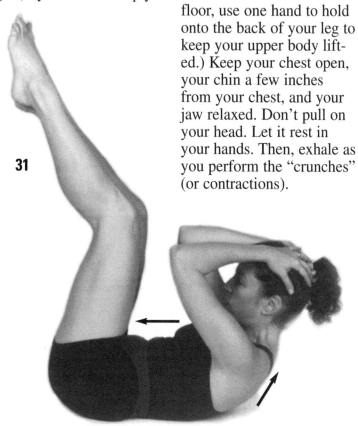

31

To increase the intensity, place your legs in as close to a 90° angle as possible. The lower your feet are (without touching the floor), the harder the exercise will be. Think of pressing "down" into the floor with your pelvis as you contract.

Part G

Cool-Down

Abdominal Stretch

32. Lie on your back with your entire body flat on the floor. Reach your arms overhead and hold a nice long stretch from end to end.

32

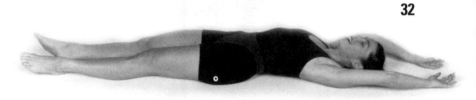

32a

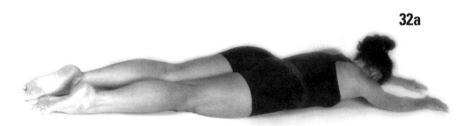

32a. Then, roll onto your stomach. Bend your arms, place your forearms on the floor, lift your head and chest, and rest on your elbows (not pictured). Look straight ahead with your back gently arched and belly button lifted off the floor. You should feel a stretch in your abdomen. Breathe and hold stretch for 20 to 30 seconds.

Back, Calf, & Hamstring Stretch

33. Place your hands by your chest, bend your knees, and pull your hips to your heels. Place the balls of your feet on the floor and rest your hips on your heels to stretch your calves and back.

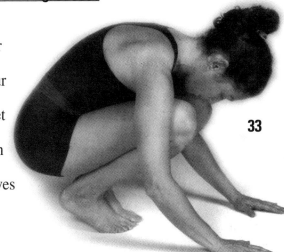

33

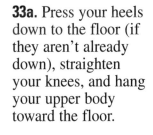

33a. Press your heels down to the floor (if they aren't already down), straighten your knees, and hang your upper body toward the floor.

33a

109

33b. Shake out your head, then bend your knees, and roll up slowly, one vertebra at a time, to standing in perfect alignment. Make sure you focus as you come up so you don't get dizzy.

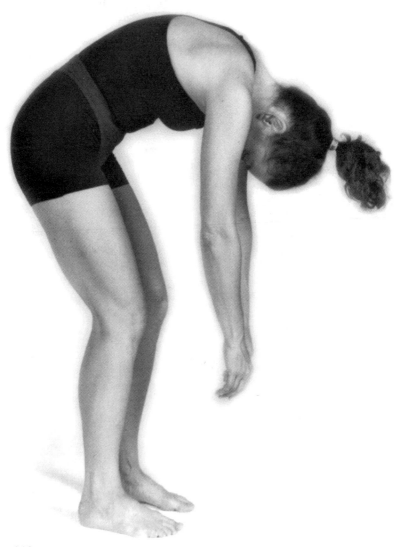

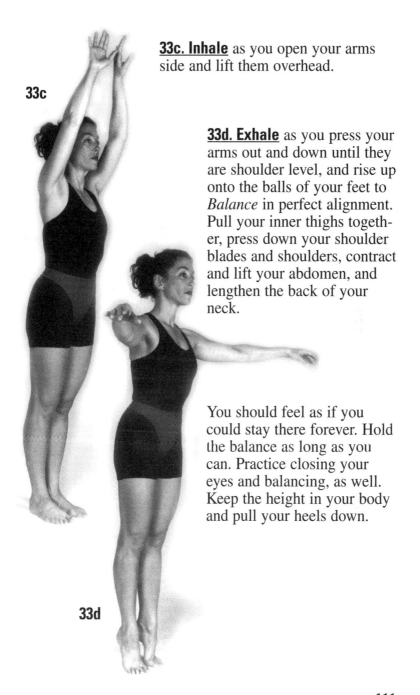

33c. <u>Inhale</u> as you open your arms side and lift them overhead.

33d. <u>Exhale</u> as you press your arms out and down until they are shoulder level, and rise up onto the balls of your feet to *Balance* in perfect alignment. Pull your inner thighs together, press down your shoulder blades and shoulders, contract and lift your abdomen, and lengthen the back of your neck.

You should feel as if you could stay there forever. Hold the balance as long as you can. Practice closing your eyes and balancing, as well. Keep the height in your body and pull your heels down.

That's it.
GREAT JOB!
See you tomorrow.

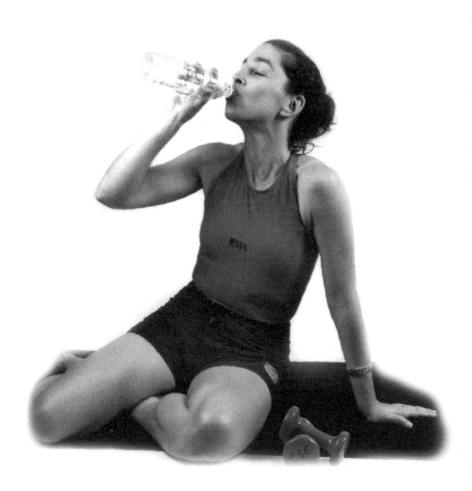

Daily Fitness Log for _____

(month)

Weight _____ **Pant size** _____ **Dress size** _____ **What changes have you noticed?**

_____

_____

(fill top part out at beginning of each month)

DATE	# mins. Tone-Up	type & # mins. Aerobic Exercise	How I ate today	How I feel today	Other relevant activities
1st					
2nd					
3rd					
4th					
5th					
6th					
7th					
8th					
9th					
10th					
11th					
12th					
13th					
14th					
15th					
16th					
17th					
18th					
19th					
20th					
21st					
22nd					
23rd					
24th					
25th					
26th					
27th					
28th					
29th					
30th					
31st					

(make copies of this page)

Answers to Quiz on page 11
and where you can find them

1.	True	chapter 1		**15.**	False	chapter 7
2.	False	chapter 1		**16.**	True	chapter 7
3.	False	chapter 1		**17.**	False	chapter 7
4.	False	chapter 1		**18.**	True	chapter 7
5.	True	chapter 1		**19.**	True	chapter 8
6.	True	chapter 2		**20.**	False	chapter 8
7.	True	chapter 4		**21.**	True	chapter 8
8.	True	chapter 4		**22.**	False	chapter 9
9.	True	chapter 4		**23.**	False	chapter 9
10.	False	chapter 5		**24.**	False	chapter 10
11.	False	chapter 5		**25.**	False	chapter 10
12.	True	chapter 6		**26.**	True	chapter 10
13.	True	chapter 5		**27.**	False	chapter 10
14.	True	chapter 7		**28.**	False	chapter 10

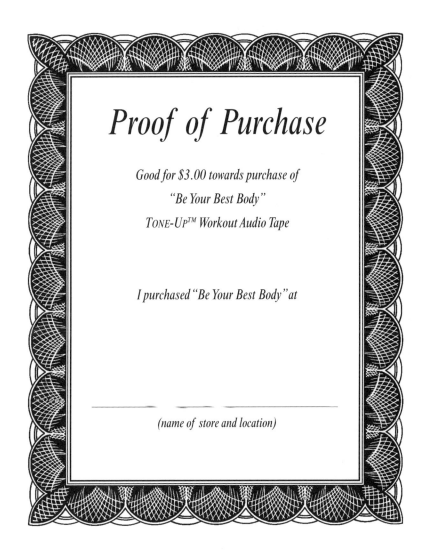

Proof of Purchase

Good for $3.00 towards purchase of
"Be Your Best Body"
TONE-UP™ Workout Audio Tape

I purchased "Be Your Best Body" at

_____

(name of store and location)

Order Form

☎ **Telephone orders:** Call (805) 898-8910.
Have your VISA or Mastercard ready.
💻 **On-line orders:** ToneUpPub@aol.com
✉ **Postal orders:** TONE-UP Publishing, Suesan Pawlitski,
P.O. Box 30058, Santa Barbara, Ca. 93130

Be Your Best Body book(s) _____ @ $12.95 = $ _____
TONE-UP Audio tape(s) _____ @ $12.95 = $ _____
Deduct $3.00 from one tape with enclosed coupon $ _____

Book & Tape Set(s) @ $22.95 = $ _____
(save $3.00)
Sales Tax: Add 7.75% for orders shipped in California. $ _____

Total $ _____
Postage and handling included.

Name: _____

Address: _____

City: _____ State: _____ Zip _____

Telephone: (_____) _____

Payment:
❑ Check
❑ Credit Card: ❑ Visa ❑ Mastercard
Card number: _____
Name on Card: _____ Exp. Date: _____/_____

Where did you purchase this book? _____

Order Form

☎ **Telephone orders:** Call (805) 898-8910.
Have your VISA or Mastercard ready.
🖳 **On-line orders:** ToneUpPub@aol.com
✉ **Postal orders:** TONE-UP Publishing, Suesan Pawlitski,
P.O. Box 30058, Santa Barbara, Ca. 93130

Be Your Best Body book(s) ———— @ $12.95 = $ ————————
TONE-UP Audio tape(s) ———— @ $12.95 = $ ————————
Deduct $3.00 from one tape with enclosed coupon $ ————————

Book & Tape Set(s) @ $22.95 = $ ————————
(save $3.00)
Sales Tax: Add 7.75% for orders shipped in California. $ ————————

Total $ ————————
Postage and handling included.

Name: _____

Address: _____

City: _____ State: _____ Zip _____

Telephone: (____) _____

Payment:
❑ Check
❑ Credit Card: ❑ Visa ❑ Mastercard
Card number: _____
Name on Card: _____ Exp. Date: ____ /_____

Where did you purchase this book? _____